Treatment of Disease with Acupuncture

By

Dr. James Tin Yau So

Volume Two
of
A Complete Course in Acupuncture

Paradigm Publications Brookline, Massachusetts
1987

Treatment of Disease with Acupuncture
By
Dr. James Tin Yau So

ISBN 0-912111-08-9

Library of Congress Number 84-9478

Published by:
Paradigm Publications
44 Linden Street
Brookline, Massachusetts 02146

This book was produced and typeset using software and services provided by Textware International of Cambridge, Massachusetts.

Cover design by Herb Rich III
Calligraphy by Chun-Han Zhu

Foreword

The opportunity to work with Dr. James So in my medical office was among the most valuable experiences of my professional career. The insight with which Dr. So approached his patients was truly remarkable, and the results he achieved in the course of treatment were startling, often seriously challenging the very foundations of my medical training and belief system. I am still in contact with patients whose relief from pain and discomfort continues to this day, years after a single treatment from Dr. So. I have seen no one since who has matched his skill and compassion.

As Dr. So worked his often incredible healing feats, I soon came to regard myself more as his student than his employer. It was inevitable that, eventually, I would count myself as one of his patients, too. My plans to run the 1982 Boston Marathon had been hindered by weeks of pain in my hip. By the night before the race, simply walking was painful. It was only after a last-chance visit to Dr. So, late in the evening before the race, that relief was brought. That single treatment of Dr. So's allowed me to enter and finish a race given up for lost, and left me free of pain to this day.

This book is a treasure of Dr. So's treatments and methods, shared openly, as has always been Dr. So's custom, and with but one objective in mind: to relieve pain and suffering as effectively as possible. Though we in my medical practice often turn to Dr. So's work for guidance, it is our patients who are the true beneficiaries of its application.

It is one of the great honors of my life to have been asked by Dr. So to write this brief introduction. I am certain that with this volume, both the practitioner and the patient will wish to share the gratitude that I, and all of Dr. So's students, so often wish to express.

Thank you, Dr. So!

James P. Doyle, D.O.

Editor's Note

Treatment of Disease with Acupuncture, volume II of **A Complete Course in Acupuncture**, includes the complete texts of *The Treatment of Disease by Acupuncture* and *The Book of Acupuncture Techniques*, as published in 1977 by the New England School of Acupuncture. Originally compiled by Dr. So in 1946, and published in 1960 in Chinese, these works were designed as practical teaching guides during a time when virtually no such works were available, and were specifically intended to accompany classroom instruction. Thus, except for his in-class examples, illustrations, and inspirations, this volume, along with his *Book of Acupuncture Points*, contains virtually all the material presented by Dr. So to his students during their intensive acupuncture training under him.

Neither speculative nor philosophical, this work is first and foremost a practical guide. It represents the combined knowledge and clinical experiences of three generations of acupuncture masters, from Ching Tan An, through his student Tsang Tien Chi (Dr. So's teacher), compiled finally by an extraordinarily talented physician who was often depended upon as the sole health care provider within his community.

As with volume one of this two volume series, the editorial goal in presenting this work has been the accurate preservation of both the precision and the flavor of Dr. So's life work. Dr. So himself participated closely throughout its publication, updating, clarifying and expanding information presented in previous editions. The result of the collaboration has produced a comprehensive acupuncture and moxibustion manual, accessible as a primary text to the beginning acupuncture student, and as a clinical reference work for the seasoned professional.

The work is divided into five broad sections:

I *Origins, Principles and Basic Concepts*
II *Traditional Chinese Diagnosis*
III *Traditional Chinese Medical Theories*
IV *The Treatment of Specific Conditions*
V *Case Reports*

Parts I, II and III guide the student through the fundamentals of practical acupuncture and moxibustion techniques, the essentials of diagnosis and the basic theories of Chinese medicine. It includes sections on needle insertion and manipulation techniques, sterilization protocol, direct and indirect moxibustion application, ear acupuncture, diet therapy and pulse and tongue diagnosis.

Part IV, **The Treatment of Specific Conditions**, is the heart of the current volume, and is the clinical focus of the previous sections. It is comprised of specific, step-by-step treatments of some 126 diseases and disorders with acupuncture, moxibustion and, in certain cases, herbal medicines.

The volume concludes with twenty five case illustrations selected by Dr. So from his clinical experiences in Asia.

Indices include a general index, an index of herbal prescriptions, and an index of acupuncture points, cross referenced by page number to volume one of this series, *The Book of Acupuncture Points*.

Preface

Although the practice of acupuncture has changed considerably over the course of its long history, many of its methods and theories have remained essentially unaltered, and reflect the beliefs and practices of an ancient culture. Like many ancient sciences, acupuncture is a mixture of sophisticated practical techniques and unfounded superstitions. Unfortunately, many modern acupuncture practitioners have not been taught to distinguish between superstition and practicality, nor have they been encouraged by their teachers to examine their own methods critically. Thus, many of their techniques, and the theories that support them, have little clinical value. At best, they are simply a waste of time; at worst, they distract the acupuncturist from using more effective methods, and thereby inhibit the patient's recovery.

During the 1930's and 1940's, my teacher, Tsang Tien Chi, encouraged all acupuncturists to thoroughly examine the ancient techniques. I took my teacher's advice to heart, and, over the past 40 years, have made it my practice to save and refine only those methods that helped my patients, and to discard all those that did not. I have encouraged my own students to do the same, and not to blindly follow the ideas of past generations. Indeed, as Jesus said, when the blind lead the blind, both will stumble and fall. Only by using our own minds—the gift of our own intelligence and the power of observation—will we be able to discover for ourselves the ultimate usefulness of a particular method or theory, and in this way make a truly valuable contribution to the development of acupuncture.

Of course, many of the old superstitions and methods have already fallen into disuse. Through our understanding of the importance of hygiene and disease transmission, for example, we no longer warm the needle in our mouth prior to insertion, as is suggested in some of the old classics. We no longer observe the prohibition against the use of moxa on a person born in the season corresponding to the element "Metal" (autumn) for fear of melting the Metal essence by the smouldering moxa, nor do we heed the injunction against the use of needles in one born during the season of "Wood" (spring) for fear of cutting and damaging that element within them. We no longer follow the practice of dividing the body into 30 parts, each assigned a day of the month, and the ancient warning not to treat those parts on those days.

Certain old techniques have dropped from common practice because of impracticality. For example, one aspect of the Chinese Clock Theory, which assigns a specific hour of the day to each meridian, recommends treating diseased meridians only in their appointed hour. This would require round-the-clock patient care by a physician with even a moderately sized practice.

The fallacies of these few examples may seem obvious. Yet there are many methods of acupuncture, currently in vogue, with drawbacks not as immediately apparent. For example, during my many years of experience I have often experimented with the various techniques of tonification and dispersion, of which there are more than ten, and have found none of them to be effective. I believe that the tonification and dispersion methods recommended by the old books have been passed automatically from generation to generation, without any real understanding of their value. Similarly, the ancient theory and techniques of the Eight Extra Meridians, in which special combinations of "master" and "coupled" points are recommended, was developed by ancient physicians to treat people of an ancient culture. They do not address the complex illnesses and weaker bodies of modern men and women, and are therefore of limited clinical value.

These and other techniques I have found to be without merit, and many of the currently popular acupuncture theories, including many of the conceptions of "chi," to be untrue or misleading. Such findings have been corroborated by my students, who depend for their excellent clinical results more on accurate needle placement and correct stimulus of the point than on more exotic methods of questionable applicability.

I realize that my approach may seem revolutionary and non-traditional, and that many who read this material will be upset and offended by such blatant disregard for that which they hold to be true, and that which their teachers presented to them. Yet I would ask those with such feelings simply to examine, as objectively as possible, those ideas, techniques and theories. I have no objection to them per se; I simply believe them to be unnecessary.

All the methods presented in this book have been proven to be effective and dependable, having been developed through observation of their effects on my own patients. Those techniques that helped relieve pain and illness, I incorporated into my practice, taught to my students, and now offer to you in this volume; those that did not, regardless of historical origin or current popularity, I have abandoned.

The use of techniques based on superstitious beliefs is like a bottle gourd or buffalo's horn: the farther you penetrate, the narrower and darker the path becomes. Such practices bind one like a strong rope, and inhibit one's freedom of thought and action. It is my hope that today's acupuncturists will stop using such methods, and will free themselves from the bottle gourd and cut their shackles. A bright future will then be a certainty, as their skills improve and more and more people are helped.

Contents

—Part I—
Origins, Principles, Basic Concepts

—Part II—
Traditional Chinese Diagnosis

—Part III—
Traditional Chinese Medical Theories

Alphabetic List of Treatments

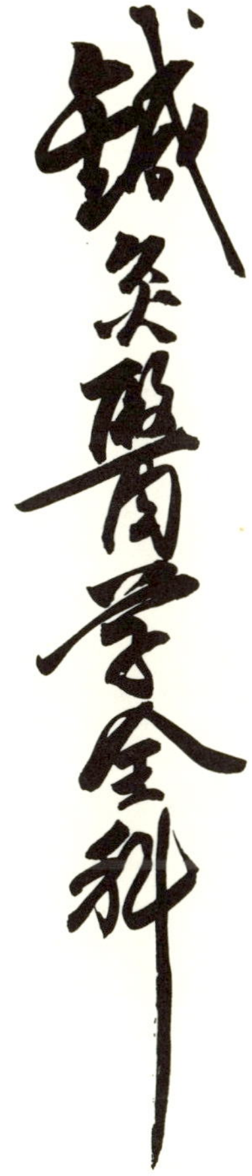

I

Origins, Principles, Basic Concepts

Chapter One Introduction

1.1 *The Origin of Acupuncture and Moxibustion*

Some suggest that the ancient Chinese invented acupuncture and moxibustion accidentally. I think it is a kind of revelation from God.

That acupuncture and moxibustion were invented by the Chinese is undoubtedly true. The exact date of their invention, however, is hard to ascertain. They were first described in the *Huang Ti Nei Ching*, a book recording the conversations between the legendary Emperor Huang Ti and Chi Po, a reknowned doctor of the time. If in fact acupuncture was practiced at the time of Huang Ti, then it must have existed for at least 5,000 years. Indeed, this conclusion was later corroborated during my visits to the acupuncturists in South Korea, where I was told that acupuncture was introduced from China to Korea 3,000 years ago.

However, according to the history of Chinese literature, the *Huang Ti Nei Ching* was a work of the period of the Warring States (403-201 B.C.E.). Thus, either the work was written at Huang Ti's time and its publication postponed until the period of the Warring States, or it was written by a later author who used the name of Huang Ti. Although there is some doubt as to the real date of the origin of this work, and of the precise date of the beginnings of acupuncture, it is clear that it has come to its present perfection as a way of medical treatment through grad- ual improvement over several thousand years.

A Brief Chronology of Chinese Medicine

ca. 1600—ca. 1100 B.C.E. The *Shang Dynasty*, with its capital city at *Yin*, is the earliest archaeologically documented period in Chinese history. Although archaeological digs in this city have not produced significant medical records, the discovery here of needle-like instruments made of jade suggests that acupuncture had been in practice as early as the Stone Age. During the later years of the *Shang*, Chi Tze, a government official, escaped the ruthless Emperor Chou, and, with a group of people from China, settled in neighboring Korea, thus introducing Chinese medicine to that country.

ca. 1100—256 B.C.E. The *Chou Dynasty*. A book named *Chou Li* is written during this time, recording the presence of four kinds of doctors: the "Food Doctor," the "Disease Doctor," the "Skin Doctor" and the "Animal Doctor." Although acupuncture is not mentioned specifically, it is possible that it was included in the "Disease Doctor" category. Also possible is that acupuncture had not yet developed to a stage at which it was widely practiced alone to treat diseases.

770—256 B.C.E. The *Eastern Chou Dynasty*. This period was a time of great internal strife; the Emperor was feeble and there was general disorder in the land. During this time, China was divided into many small kingdoms. In one such kingdom lived an eminent acupuncturist named Pin Cherk. He is credited with bringing acupuncture to the attention of the public by having had the fortune of reviving a prince of the Quirk Kingdom who had suddenly fainted and collapsed as though dead.

221—206 B.C.E. The *Chin Dynasty*. The acupuncturist Wong Po Mi writes a book called the *Chia Yi Ching*. This important work includes the names of the points, detailed methods for body measurement to aid in point location, discussions of proper needling depths, and explanations of the use of moxa in the treatment of disease. It is considered among the most important works in classical acupuncture literature. Emperor Shi Huang Ti reigned terror on scholars during this period, killing many and burning scrolls and other documents. The official Shyu Fu, cleverly playing upon the Emperor's desire for immortality, tells him of herbs growing somewhere in the Eastern Islands that may be used to prolong life. Shyu Fu is thereby ordered to travel to these Eastern Islands with 3,000 young people, in great ships, to collect specimens. He never returned, and thus escaped oppressive rule while introducign Chinese medicine to Japan.

206 B.C.E.**—25** C.E. The *Former Han Dynasty*. The *Huang Ti Nei Ching* is discovered, outlining the 14 meridians and referring to the existence of 365 acupuncture points (though listing only about 100 of those points by name). Many of the methods of treatment described in the *Huang Ti Nei Ching*, considered superstitious and/or unreliable, have been altered or discarded over the centuries.

25—220 The *Later Han Dynasty* is a period of considerable advance in traditional Chinese medicine. Medical formulae combining herbs and acupuncture become popular. The *Nan Ching* is published anonymously, though it was later doubtfully ascribed to Pin Cherk, who lived nearly 8 centuries earlier.

589—618 The *Sui Dynasty.* A full figure diagram of a man, with the acupuncture points circled and named, is conceived. Though fraught with inaccuracies, with point locations often contradicting the descriptions in the books, these diagrams allowed the codification of clinical information, which was destined to be refined and corrected as it was passed down from generation to generation.

618—906 The *Tang Dynasty.* Sun Sz Miao writes the *Chien Ching Fong*. This work further refines the practice of acupuncture by classifying the points according to diseases for which they are effective. Also introduced is the notion of *Ah Si* points (points reactive to pressure, not necessarily lying on meridians) and descriptions of treatment methods utilizing them to reduce pain.

960—1127 The *Sung Dynasty.* This is a golden period in the development of acupuncture. The successful treatment of the Emperor with acupuncture stimulates a royal decree to re-examine the points and meridians and to compile new diagrams. The famous "Bronze Man" statue is cast by Wang Wei Yi, and shows the meridians and the acupuncture points with an accuracy previously unavailable (the statue is now in the National Museum of Japan, in Tokyo, where it was taken by the Japanese during the Ching dynasty occupation.

1127—1279 The *Southern Sung Dynasty.* Two important books are published during this time: *Emergency Methods* of Si Nien, examining the use of moxa in emergency cases, and *Tzi San Ching*, of Wang Su Chuen, which names 360 acupuncture points.

1279—1366 The *Yuen Dynasty* The Mongol rule China. Fu Bi Lit, a state official, writes the book *Chin Lan Shun Ching*. The doctor Hua Po Yen redraws the meridians and points for the general public from the Bronze Statue. Ma Tan Yang publishes *Twelve Points of Stars*.

1368—1644 The *Ming Dynasty.* Acupuncture and moxibustion are quite common now. The books *A Complete Book on Acupuncture and Moxibustion* by Hsu Ting Yui, and *Shen Ying Ching* by Chen Hui are published, as well as another "complete" book on acupuncture and moxibustion by Yang Chi Chou.

1644—1911 The *Ching Dynasty.* During the latter part of the Ching dynasty, China opens its doors to trade with foreign countries. The missionaries who followed the traders cause a great deal of enmity among the Chinese people. A group of kung fu practitioners, the *Yee Wo*, tell the ruler that their practice had achieved magical proportions, and that their bodies can resist metal weapons. They are thus allowed to drive the foreigners from their land, and to kill the missionaries, foreign visitors and emmissaries. This insurgence, the *Boxer Rebellion*, is put down by the combined armies of the U.S., Britain, France, Italy and Germany, whose armies take Peiking on August 16, 1900. It is during this time that the Japanese steal the Bronze Man statue, and place it in a museum in Tokyo. Although acupuncture enjoys widespread popularity, few significant works are completed during this time. By royal instruction, a medical textbook is compiled, in which only a small portion is devoted to acupuncture. A French diplomat, George Soulie De Morant, sees the effectiveness of acupuncture when, while strolling along the street, he witnesses the revival of a fainted man with acupuncture. His subsequent request to learn acupuncture, and his translation of acupuncture texts into French, makes this medical science available to European students.

1911 marks the beginning of the Republic of China. Of the many famous acupuncturists in Kiang Su province during this time, one, Ching Tan An, revolutionizes the traditional methods, and founds a school devoted to the study of acupuncture. Tsang Tien Chi, my teacher, was one of Ching Tan An's students. Contemporary acupuncturists are quite proud of being one of Tsang's students, or of being a student of one of his students; I also feel quite fortunate to have had the opportunity to study with him.

1.2 *The Healing Principles of Acupuncture and Moxibustion*

Acupuncture — the insertion of needles into points on the body's surface — is a method of mechanical stimulation of the body. Moxibustion — the burning of the herb *Artemisia vulgaris* on the points — is a method of heat stimulation. Because neither technique uses any form of medication, both may be considered physical therapy.

Recently a Western acupuncturist made the following statement:

> The human body is an electronic device and the nerves inside are its electric wires. The brain is the main electric generator. Electric waves travel from the main generator and are distributed according to the needs of the various organs. This goes on constantly, and the health of the body is maintained. On the other hand, if any of the internal organs have an abnormality in the electric supply, through weakened, oversensitive or disturbed nerves, a disease will be produced.

There is some validity in the above statement. Each acupuncture point is regarded by the acupuncturist as a site of reaction. The stimulation of these sites with needle or moxa will activate the nerve there, and generate an electric wave that will reach the organ regulated by it. This, in fact, is the objective of acupuncture and moxibustion.

In my 40 years of clinical experience, I have found that the nerves do indeed have the characteristic ability to respond in this way to acupuncture and moxibustion treatment. The belief that the use of needles or moxa has the potential to damage the nerves is unfounded; in fact, quite the opposite is true. Their use over the course of several treatments can cure such conditions as nerve spasm and paralysis by restoring normal nerve function.

Those not educated in the application of acupuncture often believe that the therapeutic effectiveness of these techniques is limited to but a few diseases and disorders. However, the combined use of acupuncture and moxibustion can heal nearly 80 percent of all diseases, especially those not cured by any other type of medicine. If this were not true, traditional Chinese medicine would not have survived in these modern days of advanced medical science.

1.3 *Basic Concepts: Meridians and Acupuncture Points*

1.3.1 Meridians

Although the precise nature of meridians has yet to be determined by modern scientific investigation, it is helpful to think of them as the routes of the nerve fibers. The body has 14 main meridians. Each of the six solid organs (heart, liver, spleen, lung, pericardium, and kidney) and the six hollow organs (gallbladder, stomach, large intestine, small intestine, bladder, and triple warmer*) has a meridian with which it is associated. In addition, there is a meridian traversing the middle of the front of the body (known as the Conception Vessel), and one traversing the middle of the back of the body (known as the Governing Vessel).

1.3.2 Points

Points refer to the sites on the surface of the skin where stimulation by either needles or moxa elicits a response from the underlying nerve. They are located in depressions, grooves and pits, and between or on top of muscles and bones. Stimulation of the points lying along a particular meridian has a curative effect on the organ of that meridian, as well as on the other meridians.

The 14 meridians contain 365 points, of which approximately 200 are commonly used. In addition, nearly 100 points not located on the meridians have been discovered whose curative effects are specific to one or two disorders. There are approximately 20 of these so-called "extra points" in common use.

Since all points are not equally effective for the condition being treated, choosing the correct point to maximize therapeutic effect requires great skill and experience.

---

*According to Chinese medicine, the triple warmer refers to the nerve plexus between the solid organs and hollow organs, and also includes the lymphatic system.

Chapter Two
The Practice of Acupuncture

2.1 *The Physiological Basis of Needle Application*

Three basic physiological effects are evident with the application of needles: *stimulation, inhibition,* and *diversion.*

Stimulation: Needles have a stimulating effect on weakened or paralyzed areas of the body. If the sensory or motor nerves are paralyzed, needles can restore their normal functions, thus strengthening and reviving weakened internal organs.

Inhibition: During infection, dilation of the blood vessels results in excessive blood in the tissue, causing inflammation. Needles can help relieve and restrict these effects, in addition to assisting in the curing of the disease. If the sensory organs are oversensitive and painful, or if the motor nerves are over-active, thereby causing spasm, needles can have a calming and relieving effect. Needles can also have a sedative effect on overactive digestive organs, relieving such conditions as vomiting and diarrhea.

Diversion: Needles inserted into some part of a diseased area, thus stimulating the nerve endings, can divert the pathway of the circulation of the blood. For example, if there is excess blood in the brain, stimulation of the distal nerve endings will dilate the capillaries at the point of stimulation, while at the same time causing constriction of the vessels in the brain. Where internal systems have excessive blood or inflammation, needles can be inserted into the outer or superficial areas of the body in order to divert the circulation elsewhere.

2.2 *Needles: Tools of the Trade*

In ancient times, acupuncturists used nine different kinds of needles, some shaped like arrows, some like knives. The earliest were made of jade. These were regarded as too thick and cumbersome for the precise work of the acupuncturist, and later practitioners developed the use of bamboo needles, sharpened to fine points to prevent them from breaking.

When iron and steel were developed, these became the materials used to manufacture needles. Although a distinct advancement over stone and bamboo, early metal needles were, by modern standards, quite thick, and were easily stained and broken. The fine, durable, flexible, and hard needles used today were not developed until after World War Two, and were made possible by the introduction of stainless steel in needle manufacturing.

It is important to note that acupuncture needles are entirely different from needles used for sewing and injections; they are considerably thinner, and their points are shaped in such a way as to allow them to be inserted through the skin with a minimum of discomfort to the patient.

2.2.1 Needle Size

In Hong Kong, 1/2 inch to 2 1/2 inches in length is considered a sufficient size range for needle length; in this country, needles of up to 4 inches in length are commonly used. The choice of needle length should be determined by the acupuncture point that is to be needled.

In ancient times, and as recently as 100 years ago in China, needles one foot in length, with the diameter of a small chopstick, were used during the winter months, when heavy clothing had to be penetrated before the skin could be reached. The thickest gauge needles in current use are 20 gauge in diameter. These are used rarely, however, since their thickness contributes to making acupuncture therapy unnecessarily painful, as well as increasing the risk of infection. The most common needle diameters used today range from 28 to 32 gauge; needles smaller than 32 gauge make skin penetration more difficult. For needles under 1 inch in length, 31 gauge is the best diameter. For needles from 1 inch to 2 inches in length, 30 gauge is most appropriate. For needles from 2 inches to 4 inches in length, 28 and 29 gauge are used.

In recent years, individually pre-sterilized, disposable needles, in most sizes and gauges, have become available from Japan. Such needles are especially useful when treatment involves known or suspected exposure to such infectious diseases as hepatitis or AIDS.

2.2.2. Judging the Quality of an Acupuncture Needle

The acupuncture needle is constructed in three parts — handle, body, and point — and careful attention must be paid to the quality of construction of each. Although there are many different companies that manufacture acupuncture needles, there are certain criteria used to determine needle quality that are common to all. These involve *the degree of sharpness of the needle point, the smoothness of the needle body,* and *the overall springiness of the needle.*

Degree of Sharpness: Needles with short, blunt points are painful when inserted. Needles with very long, sharp points are easily damaged, and tend to develop a bent hook shape after being used a few times. The best needle points fall in between these two extremes.

Smoothness of the Needle Body: The body of the needle must be absolutely smooth, without nicks or tiny metal deposits.

Springiness: If the needle is too soft or too hard, the possibility of breakage or bending upon insertion is increased. In addition, soft needles are sometimes not strong enough to penetrate muscle tissue, and will not be able to spring back to form a straight needle shaft after being bent.

2.3 *Preliminary Considerations*

Before a single needle is inserted, careful attention must be paid to the preparation of the practitioner, to the care of his or her equipment, and to the orientation of the patient. Correct sterilization and aseptic procedures, optimum body position for the patient to receive treatment, and a thorough understanding of the techniques of needle insertion are thus essential prerequisites for safe and effective treatment.

2.3.1 Sterilization

All needles, cotton balls, gauze pads, forceps, and forceps holders must be autoclaved. Minimal requirements for correct autoclaving are 15 pounds of pressure per square inch, at 121 °C (250 °F) for 15 minutes. Longer periods of time are required if the autoclave is densely packed. Various bacteriological and chemical controls are available to help assure that adequate sterilization conditions have been achieved.

The acupuncturist must have thoroughly clean hands and nails before and after treating the patient. In addition, the area around the point must be cleaned with alcohol before needling.

While treating patients with infectious diseases such as hepatitis, syphilis or tuberculosis, be especially careful not to prick your fingers with their needles. Needles used in the treatment of these patients must be carefully segregated, and never sterilized together with other needles and equipment. Unless you have access to a gas sterilizer, use these needles for one patient only, and discard them after that patient has completed treatments. Alternatively, one should consider the use of disposable needles, mentioned previously.

2.3.2 Establishing Correct Body Positioning for Needling

Beginning acupuncturists should take special care to position their patients correctly, both for maximum therapeutic effect and patient safety. Always place yourself and the patient in such a way that the greatest stimulus of the point may be achieved in the most comfortable and efficient needling position. For example, LI-4 is best approached when sitting opposite the patient than when positioned beside the patient.

Avoid dangerous situations. For example, when inserting a needle in BL-1, near the inner canthus of the eye, the patient should be lying on his or her back, or with the head against the wall. If the head is not supported in such a way, the patient's natural reaction to move during needling might cause injury to the eye. When needling LU-11, the base of the patient's thumb, rather than the other side of the thumbnail, should be held securely to avoid cutting the skin in the event that the patient pulls the hand away when the stimulus is felt.

Thus, the patient may be required to lie down, sit, or stand depending on the point to be needled. Once the correct posture has been obtained, instruct the patient not to move. In the United States today, many acupuncturists instruct their patients to lie down for all needling procedures, regardless of the point being treated. This practice limits their ability to needle some regions of the body as effectively as possible.

2.3.3 Holding and Inserting the Needle

Needles are inserted either perpendicular to the surface of the skin; obliquely (i.e., at an angle to the skin's surface); or along the surface of the skin.

During insertion, the base of the needle handle is held with the index finger and thumb of the right hand, with the middle finger used to support the body of the needle. The middle finger should apply gentle pressure to the body of the needle, bending it in an S shape. This will have the effect of strengthening the needle, thus making insertion easier. The point to be treated is located with the left hand.

The Pressing Finger

The index finger or thumb of the acupuncturist's left hand is used to fix the point, and in this capacity is called the "pressing finger." The point of the needle is inserted next to the nail of the pressing finger.

Correct action of the pressing finger is essential for proper needle insertion. In general, the pressing finger is utilized in the following ways:

- To keep the needle stationary
- To guide the needle to the correct point
- To press the skin and keep the skin stationary
- To help prevent the patient from moving
- To make insertion easier by compressing the skin

For loose skin, to obtain a strong stimulus, and for deep insertions, the pressing finger should apply relatively greater pressure on the point.

For sensitive skin, for patients who are nervous, and for inflamed areas, the pressure of the pressing finger should be very light, the finger itself just touching the skin.

2.3.4 Areas That Are Forbidden to Needle

The following areas may not be needled:

- The spinal bulb and spinal cord
- The eyeballs
- The testicles
- GV-22 on children under eight
- Any pulse (artery) or vein
- Any internal organs

Your needle should never hit an organ (i.e., the needle should never penetrate into the body cavity); if this occurs there will be very serious consequences.

> *If the heart is hit, death in one day, the action of death is with the voice, Ah!*
>
> *If the liver is hit, death in five days, the action of death is talking.*

> *If the kidney is hit, death in six days, the action of death is sneezing.*
>
> *If the lung is hit, death in three days, the action of death is coughing.*
>
> *If the spleen is hit, death in ten days, the action of death is swallowing.*
>
> *If the gallbladder is hit, death in one and a half days, the action of death is talking.*

A needle inserted in GV-17 (''Brain Door''), will hit the brain and the patient will die immediately.

2.4 *Techniques for Penetrating the Skin*

Efficient penetration of the skin requires significant skill. Indeed, a major part of your reputation as a good acupuncturist depends upon your ability to insert the needle with the least amount of discomfort to the patient. If you are lacking in this skill, needle insertion will be unpleasant for both you and the patient, no matter how small the needle.

It is essential that the needle be sharp and straight, and that the action of the pressing finger, the application of pressure on the needle, and the direction of insertion be controlled and coordinated. In addition, the sensitivity of the patient's skin and its resistance to the needle must be understood and taken into account.

The needle is pressed through the skin using one of the insertion methods discussed below. After penetrating the skin, additional pressure is applied to the needle to insert it deeper into the flesh. When the needle point touches the nerve and the patient feels the stimulus, apply the appropriate needle manipulation technique according to the case being treated.

2.4.1 The Eight Methods for Penetrating the Skin

1) The Three Step Method: Touch the point of the needle to the skin. Press down on the needle until it penetrates the skin. This should be done relatively quickly. This method is not used on the face.

2) Slow Insertion: Touch the point of the needle to the skin. Using slow, steady pressure, press the needle until it penetrates the skin. The pressing finger should apply relatively more pressure in this method than in the previous one.

3) Faster Insertion: This technique is three times as fast the **slow insertion** method.

4) Flying Needle: This method is used for patients with very sensitive skin, and for areas of the body that, in some patients, are very muscular (i.e. lower back, upper arm, upper leg). Insert the needle as one would give an injection. Do not use the pressing finger until after the needle has been inserted.

5) Needle Flying In and Out: This method is used for bleeding the ''Well Points'' on the fingers and toes. Using the prismatic needle, puncture the point very quickly, in approximately 1/10 of a second. The patient will hardly feel anything. For PC-9, located on the tip of the middle finger, a thick (low gauge) needle is used instead of the prismatic needle.

6) Vibrating Needle: In this gentle method of insertion, the pressing finger is not used until after the needle has entered the skin. The needle is vibrated up and down on the point until it penetrates the skin. After the needle is in, add the pressing finger; otherwise, the skin will cling to the needle as it moves in and out or up and down.

7) Pressing Needle: This technique is used when treating the palm of the hand and the sole of the foot, where, although the skin is very thick, it is also very sensitive. Use a shorter and thicker needle and a great deal of pressure with the pressing finger. Penetration should be very fast. Though some pain is to be expected during insertion, if the pressing finger is not moved once the needle is under the skin, additional manipulation techniques will be almost painless.

8) Twisting Needle: Touch the skin with the needle point and then twist it in with pressure. This method is for areas and skin conditions that make insertion difficult, such as stiff skin and areas with scars.

In ancient times, some acupuncturists would ask their patients to cough, and simultaneously insert the needle. This would distract the patient, and tend to reduce the pain caused by the larger needles.

If you must treat a point on which a moxa burn is still healing, do not penetrate the scar with the needle. Rather, use the pointing finger of the left hand to pull the scar off to the side, and the middle finger as the pressing finger on the point.

2.4.2 Insertion Techniques for Deep Needling

When inserting the needle into deep acupuncture points, the muscles tend to bunch around the needle, following its movement inward. This problem can be avoided by first inserting the needle only a fraction of the distance, and then alternately withdrawing the needle a third of the distance out, and pressing it in one third again, until the desired depth has been achieved. This in-and-out effect has the property of loosening the needle. If you do not touch the nerve after penetrating the proper distance, pull the needle out a little, angle to the right or to the left, and then re-insert.

2.4.3 Depth of Insertion

Because of the wide variety of body types and patient characteristics, it is difficult to generalize about the correct depth of insertion. The insertion depth suggested should therefore always be considered an estimate. You may have to insert the needle a little deeper than the depth recommended, and you may have to try angling the needle to the left or to the right to touch the nerve correctly. Once you stimulate the nerve, do not insert the needle any deeper. The head, the neck, the chest, and the upper back house the brain, spinal cord, and viscera. A needle inserted too deeply into points in these areas might cause injury.

There is one faction of acupuncturists who will insert the needle very deeply, regardless of the area of the body in which the point is located, Another faction always uses very shallow insertion. Neither method is of the highest standard, and therefore neither should be practiced.

Remove the needle slowly. After the needle is out, press and rub the point with a cotton ball, held in the left hand, in order to close the opening left in the skin after needling.

2.4.4 Bleeding Technique

Points are bled in conditions of inflammation and/or poor circulation. There are two methods for bleeding points: one uses the prismatic needle to draw blood from the finger and toe Well points; the other uses a special bleeding needle to draw blood from the veins. Use a tourniquet to help expose the vein. Be careful not to penetrate through the vein or to bleed an artery.

2.5 Painful Needle Insertion: Causes and Remedies

2.5.1 Needle Phobia

People are often afraid of acupuncture because of their personal history with needles, and are likely to interpret *any* stimulus as being painful. It is therefore of great importance that the acupuncturist learns to insert the needle painlessly.

Explain to the patient that their previous experiences with sewing needles and hypodermics have been painful because of the size of the needles, but that acupuncture needles are much smaller than these ordinary needles. Explain also that it is usually the hands or fingers, the more sensitive parts of the body, that are pricked by sewing needles, and that most acupuncture points are not as sensitive as these areas.

2.5.2 Improper Use of the Pressing Finger

Needling may be painful if the pressing finger moves during insertion, is too far from the point before insertion, is pressed down too hard or not hard enough, or is lifted up and then pressed down again. Remember not to remove the pressing finger after the needle has been inserted.

2.5.3 Dull or Crooked Needles

The point of the needle may not be sharp enough, and may have developed a small hook. To repair an acupuncture needle, you will need a three-fold magnifying glass with 10x magnification; an Arkansas whetstone; and some sewing machine oil. Put 1-3 drops of sewing machine oil on the stone. Holding the lower part of the needle's handle, rub the point back and forth against the stone's surface, while simultaneously rotating the needle between the thumb and first finger. Check the needle's sharpness with the magnifying glass. When the point has the right amount of sharpness, burnish it with golden sandpaper. Wrap a corner of the paper around the point and twist the needle back and forth while drawing it in and out.

To straighten a needle that has become curved, and is shaped like a crescent moon, hold it with the tip pointing toward the ground. Starting at the base of the needle body, draw the thumb and forefinger along the needle body while pressing with those fingers.

2.5.4 The Fingers Used for Insertion are Weak

If the acupuncturist's fingers are not strong enough, several attempts may be required before penetration of the skin is accomplished. This may be remedied by practicing any of the following methods for finger strengthening.

Method I: Using an old book, begin by inserting the needle through 2 pages at a time. When this becomes easy, add more pages. When you can easily insert the needle through a thickness of 1/2 to 1 inch, your fingers should have gained enough strength to practice acupuncture.

Method II: Tie an orange-sized bundle of cotton tightly with some string. Insert the needle through this ball repeatedly, until insertion is easy. Then tie it with more string, and practice with the needle again until insertion is easy.

Method III: Fold a rubber sponge tightly and bind it with rubber bands. Insert needles in this home-made rubber ball until insertion can be done with ease. Add more rubber bands, and continue practicing until insertion is easy. When you have destroyed two sponges, your fingers should be strong enough to practice.

2.5.5 A Technique for Training the Chi to Improve Insertion Techniques

This technique should be done in the early morning or early evening in a quiet place.

Sit on the floor, or on any flat space, in such a way that wind does not blow against your face. Sit straight, in a lotus position, with chest erect, and the hands folded and resting in your lap. Inhale through the nose, completely expanding the lungs, hold the breath for a second and then exhale through the mouth, completely emptying the lungs. Rest a moment before the next inhalation; the slower this is done the better. Count each breath you take, to help quiet your inner mind. Continue for 20 to 30 minutes. Performed daily, your body's chi will become much more powerful.

2.5.6 Additional Causes of Painful Insertion

Finally, one should be aware of the following conditions, which may contribute to pain from needle insertion:

- The needle is inserted through the surface of the skin, but not past the pain receptive area under the skin;
- The needle has come out from the point, and is then reinserted into the same spot;
- The patient has very tough skin, making acupuncture more painful;
- The patient is extremely sensitive;
- After inserting the needle, the patient moves, and thus bends the needle;
- The needle has hit a vein, causing undue pain.

2.6 *The Reaction of the Point: The Stimulus*

When the needle touches the nerve, the patient will describe an electric-like sensation, or a sensation of soreness, dullness, aching, or heaviness. This is the reaction of the nerve. It is very important for the acupuncturist to obtain this reaction, for without it, all work will be in vain. Some points react slightly, while some react very strongly to the needle; in all cases, though, some reaction must be obtained.

Occasionally, the acupuncturist will encounter a patient in whom no points elicit reactions. The ancient book instructs that if you meet this kind of patient, insert a needle in CV-6; if there is still no reaction to needling, the patient cannot be cured. Five direct moxa on GV-20 may also be tried in an attempt to restore reactivity. As a last resort, substitution of direct moxa for needles may be attempted.

Degree of Stimulus: The degree of stimulus to be obtained is determined by a number of factors, including patient body type; sex and age of the patient; type of case being treated; and area of the body on which the points lie.

In general, a **light stimulus** is most appropriate for children and young adults; for thin and/or weak patients; for patients who are nervous; and for points on the face, hands, and on the soles of the feet.

Strong stimulus should be used for patients with a lot of fatty tissue; for older and middle-aged patients; for patients with strong bodies; and for cases of arthritis, neuritis, numbness, and loss of consciousness.

2.7 *Needle Manipulation Techniques*

In the ancient books, a number of esoteric methods are described for needle manipulation for tonification and dispersion (adding energy to or taking energy from points). For example, it is said that tonification or dispersion may be achieved by the direction in which the acupuncturist rotates the needle after insertion. However, after many years of practice, I have found that what is most important is obtaining the correct stimulation.

The following are methods to be used to stimulate the points after the needle has been inserted.

Single Stimulus: Insert the needle in the point, stimulate the nerve once, and then remove the needle. This is a relatively light stimulation.

Twisting Needle: Stimulate the nerve with the needle, and then rotate the needle to the right and to the left. This will stimulate the point more than a single stimulus. This technique may also be used on head points, where it is sometimes difficult to touch the nerve correctly.

Bird Pecking: After touching the nerve, manipulate the needle up and down, like a bird pecking the ground. This will result in very strong stimulation.

Skin Needle: For this technique, the needle should not penetrate the skin, but should lightly touch the skin's surface several times. This technique is used for infants, whose skin is very sensitive, and for minor ailments in children. Stimulating the free nerve endings on the skin in these young patients is sufficient to trigger the deeper nerves. *Do not use this technique in cases of convulsions or high fevers.*

Laying Needle: After the needle is inserted and you have obtained the correct reaction, leave the needle in the point for 20 to 30 minutes. For some chronic cases and severe pain problems this technique can be very effective.

Heavy Pricking: On either a single point or over a wide area, prick the skin's surface repeatedly with the needle. This technique can be used to bleed a point (like *Faht Jei*), to help relieve the itching of ringworm, and to stimulate sensations in numb patches of skin. Avoid the use of the instrument known as the seven-star hammer.

Chapter Three
The Practice of Moxibustion

Heat applied to certain parts of the body, specifically to acupuncture points, has been shown since ancient times to be effective in ridding disease and increasing the general level of health. Because of this, Chinese physicians have developed the clinical art of moxibustion, which, when used in conjunction with the application of needles, greatly increases the potential for effective treatment of a wide variety of diseases.

3.1 *Moxa*

The substance used for moxibustion is obtained from the leaves of the plant *Artemisia vulgaris* of the family Compositae, a small plant that grows wild and abundantly on mountains and in fields. The lower surface of the leaf has a layer of white hair or fur, which, when dried, becomes the spongy, tissue-like material called moxa.

Moxa is harvested just before the fifth of Chinese May (June in Western calendars). The plant is cut down, and the leaves stripped from the branches and allowed to dry in the sun. The big, thick leaves are said to contain the most powerful healing properties. When the leaves have dried, they are put in a cloth bag (burlap is often used), and aged for two to three years. The quality of the moxa changes daily during this time, and it is commonly believed that the longer the moxa has been allowed to mature, the more potent its medicinal properties. Mencius said: "For a disease of seven years duration, you should use moxa that is at least three years old."

After aging, the leaves are pounded with mortar and pestle, and then cleaned by rubbing against a sieve until the resulting substance is as soft as cotton, and has become fairly white in color. Particles that penetrate the sieve, including the ash-colored portions of the upper side of the leaves, are considered debris, and are discarded. The more time spent in rubbing, the whiter and more pure the moxa.

Since most acupuncturists live in the city, harvesting and processing their own moxa is obviously impractical. It is more convenient to purchase moxa from an herb shop. To do this, one must be able to recognize the highest quality moxa. The lighter, whiter the color, the purer the moxa, and the less pain it causes when used directly on the skin. Moxa that is half white and half black is of medium quality. Moxa that is more black than white is not of good quality; very dark moxa is of very bad quality. Moxa that is not black, but a yellow or green color, is less than one year old and should not be used.

Properly aged moxa has a rich, somewhat mellow fragrance. New moxa (moxa with yellow or green coloring) smells like cut grass.

When high quality moxa is squeezed, it will spring back slightly, somewhat like a rubber sponge. Bad quality moxa will not spring back.

3.2 *The Physiological Effects of Moxibustion*

According to Chinese medical texts, moxa is warm, bitter, and non-poisonous, and may be effectively used to achieve the following therapeutic effects:

- to increase the circulation of blood and chi in the twelve meridians
- to remove cold sensations
- to remove *supp*
- to lift the spirit
- to help muscles heal
- to keep the uterus warm during pregnancy
- to kill tapeworms and intestinal worms when taken internally
- to help revive dying yang

When burned directly on the skin, moxa has the advantage of being a non-poisonous fuel. Although there is the initial pain felt as a result of the minor burn on the skin, when the heat is removed, the residual pain is minimal. Further, moxa has a germicidal effect, and therefore the risk of infection after burning is minimized. When moxa burns do get infected, the infection is contained at the site of the burn, and does not spread to form an ulcer. This germicidal effect is also evident in the action of moxa against germs on the skin surface, and in superficial wounds of the muscles.

Japanese doctors have heated egg-sized portions of moxa under a mercury trough, in order to measure its thermal characteristics. The heat obtained under such circumstances measured 360 °F. They have also used moxa on rabbits. From these experiments they have found that moxa will increase the number of blood cells, especially white cells, will dilate the blood vessels, increase blood pressure, raise body temperature, promote blood and lymphatic circulation, and increase the absorption of secretory materials.

Three specific physiological effects are evident with the application of moxa on the skin: *distal stimulation, direct stimulation,* and *reflective stimulation.*

Distal Stimulation: This effect supports the ancient saying, "for a disease in the upper part, treat the lower part." For example, if there is a disease in the head or thorax, we can apply moxa to the hands or the feet.

Direct Stimulation: Moxa may be applied directly to the affected part to relieve pain, stop inflammation, reduce swelling, and relieve paralysis.

Reflective Stimulation: If the internal viscera are diseased, moxa can be applied to the sympathetic nerves on the back. It will be reflected inside and heal the disease.

There are two ways to apply moxa: *directly* or *indirectly.* In ancient practice, moxa was applied only directly. Direct moxa is considerably more effective than indirect moxa, especially in life-threatening and emergency situations, and in stubborn, chronic diseases. In addition, the application of direct moxa has the ability to change the functions of the solid organs.

However, direct moxa is quite painful, and will leave a scar. For this reason, modern acupuncturists have devised a variety of methods of moxibustion that protect the skin from scarring and reduce discomfort. These include applying moxa on a piece of ginger, burning moxa on the handles of the needles, and burning moxa in an instrument which is then placed over a piece of gauze. All these indirect methods are useful, although their therapeutic effectiveness is limited to lighter ailments. To be a good acupuncturist, one should understand every technique of acupuncture and moxibustion, and the best method to apply in each case.

3.3 *Direct Moxa*

Moxa applied directly to the skin and burnt to the skin's surface is a powerful and penetrating form of heat therapy. Direct moxa is recommended for both chronic and acute conditions, and in the treatment of overcooling conditions of the body. It is essential in the treatment of such diseases as tuberculosis, scrofula, cancers or tumors, neuralgia, cramps, numbness, anorexia, inflammation of the uterus, asthma, gonorrhea, chronic inflammation, beri-beri, pain in joints, rheumatism, and arthritis. Direct moxa is unsuitable for patients with fevers (except in cases of tuberculosis with fever), cerebral congestion, high blood pressure, and in cases of apoplexy accompanied by a strong pulse.

Direct moxa speeds up the therapeutic process, and quickly eliminates pain. Do not worry about the patient refusing direct moxibustion. Most patients are more concerned with recovering quickly than with the methods used to achieve that recovery. Do not be concerned with the small amount of pain direct moxa causes, nor with the small scar it leaves. The procedure will often significantly speed recovery, and perhaps be instrumental in eliminating the need for surgery.

Before applying direct moxa, explain the process to the patient in such a way that they will agree to its application.

In ancient times, acupuncturists used a magnifying glass to get the "fire" from the sun to light the moxa, and felt that this was the only non-poisonous way to ignite it. This is not really true. The other material only starts the moxa fire and what is then burning is only the moxa. Therefore you should be able to use any method to light moxa, without worrying about contamination.

3.3.1 The Shape and Size of Direct Moxa

The size of moxa should be determined by the patient's ability to withstand the discomfort of the burn, the type of case being treated, and the health of the body.

Prescriptions for direct moxa call for the following sizes: chestnut and peanut size (the largest); yellow bean and red bean sizes; and green been size, 1/2 rice grain size and sesame seed size (the smallest sizes used).

In all sizes, moxa should be rolled tightly and spherically Tight, hard moxa has more penetrating power, and the spherical shape will leave the least disfiguring scar. Put an appropriate amount of moxa between the tips of the thumb and first finger, roll it into a small ball, and then roll it along the side of the first finger, pressing with some force with the thumb. Never roll back to the finger tip. Use the other hand to pick up the moxa and put it on the point.

Ancient people used garlic juice to keep the moxa from falling off the point. Now we use Vaseline or Vicks Vapo-Rub. This is applied in a thin layer on the point, and the moxa applied on top. After burning each moxa, use a cotton ball to remove the ash. After burning the necessary number of moxas, apply Vicks Vapo-Rub to the scar, and cover it with a band-aid to prevent irritation.

3.3.2 Minimizing the Pain Caused by Direct Moxa

While the moxa is burning, rub the surrounding skin lightly with the fingernail to help lessen the pain. If the patient is overly frightened of the pain, use one of the following techniques:

1) Apply moxa, and when the patient feels that it is too painful, remove it. Apply another piece of moxa, again removing it when the patient reports that the pain is unbearable. Repeating this procedure, you will notice that with each application, the patient will be able to withstand the moxa for a longer time. Continue in this manner until the patient is able to withstand having the moxa burned all the way down to the surface of the skin. Consider the first moxa to be burned all the way down as the first moxa of the treatment.

2) Use a very small piece of moxa for the first moxa; the patient will feel only a little pain. Progressively increase the size of the moxa until it is of the recommended size for the case being treated. The first correctly sized moxa should be considered the first moxa of the treatment.

It has been suggested that local anesthetic injections be employed to eliminate the pain caused by direct moxa. If this were done, the nerves would be numb and unable to react to the stimulus; the burning procedure would thus be in vain.

For points that need to be repeatedly burned, burn the moxa on top of the previous scar. To minimize the pain of burning moxa on a scar which has been scratched off, cover the scar with a piece of garlic about 1/16 inch in thickness, and apply the moxa on top of the garlic. After applying moxa, apply mercurochrome to the scar.

3.3.3 Areas Unsuitable for Direct Moxa

Do not apply moxa

- around the eyes
- around the testicles
- on pulse or vein
- on GV-15 and GV-16 (to avoid hurting the spinal cord and risking muteness)

The number of moxas applied to the general area around the heart or on the abdomen of women over five months pregnant should be limited. Avoid burning too much moxa on the lower abdomen and on the back of the head. Finally, use direct moxa sparingly on the hands and feet.

3.3.4 Precautions to Take After Applying Direct Moxa

After undergoing moxa therapy, the patient should be given the following recommendations:

- Do not eat immediately after treatment, (although it is important to eat after a short interval);
- Rest for some time;
- Abstain from sex for 24 hours;
- Do not let the cold wind blow on the body;
- Avoid cold foods.

If the scar is inflamed, the patient should avoid eating ginger, which would make the sore more itchy and eventually more ugly.

3.4 *Indirect Moxa*

The date of the invention of indirect moxibustion is unknown. It is used for patients who are afraid of the pain caused by direct moxa, for those who want to avoid scarring, and, in general for all light ailments.

3.4.1 Indirect Moxa with Ginger

This technique initially involved using only a very small piece of ginger between the skin and the moxa. This alleviated some pain from the burning process. However, blisters would still form, concomitant with scars. Later, this method was changed, and we now use a piece of ginger the thickness of two 25 cent pieces, 1 inch wide and 11/2 inches long. Put the moxa on the piece of ginger, light it, and wait until it burns down to the ginger, and the bottom side of the ginger feels hot to the touch. Apply the ginger to the appropriate point. If it is too hot for the patient, remove it from the skin for 1-2 seconds, and then re-apply. The best way to use indirect moxa by ginger is when there are two points that need moxa, and you can switch the hot piece of ginger from one point to the other. Continue application until the ginger is no longer hot. This is a quick way to apply indirect moxa, and it prevents blistering. It is about one third as strong as direct moxa. A piece of ginger can be used only once. If you need to heat several points, prepare 2-3 pieces at a time. When the first piece of ginger is hot enough to use, light the second piece.

3.4.2 Indirect Moxa with Garlic

Peel the garlic and pound until soft and mushy. Apply the garlic to the area that needs moxa in a small mountain or pyramid shape. Burn 30 to 50 peanut sized rolls of moxa on top of the garlic; the whole area should become very hot. This technique can be used on carbuncles that are just forming, or on areas that are just beginning to develop an inflammation. When applying the moxa to an area which is initially painful, apply it until there is no more pain. When applying the moxa to an area which is not painful initially, apply it until it becomes painful.

3.4.3 Indirect Moxa with Salt

This is the only method used when treatment of the point CV-8, the umbilicus, is called for, since needles may not be inserted at that point.

If the umbilicus is deep, fill it with salt to the level of the skin. Burn the moxa on the salt. The salt will transmit the heat to the entire umbilicus. If the umbilicus is shallow, you can apply moxa directly on the skin, although the use of salt is most effective.

3.4.4 Indirect Moxa with Chinese Herb Powder

Mix powdered *Fu Tzu* (Aconite) with hot water to form a paste. Shape the paste into a small cookie and apply to the diseased area. Moxa is then burned on top of this herb until the inside of the diseased area feels very hot. This is good for a "cold ulcer," a condition in which a post-surgical wound will not heal and continues to drain liquid daily.

3.4.5 Indirect Moxa with Moxa Instrument

The moxa instrument was developed in Japan. Moxa is put inside the instrument, lit and burned until the instrument feels sufficiently hot. The instrument is then rubbed on the appropriate points, over which a piece of gauze has been placed. If the patient feels that the instrument is too hot, another layer of gauze may be added. The heat of the instrument should be adjusted for each particular patient's skin. Many kinds of moxa instruments are available, including a kind of tea filter used in this country that is suitable for indirect moxa.

3.4.6 Moxa Applied to the Handle of the Needle

In this method, moxa is rolled in paper to form a cigar-shaped pole, 3/4 of an inch in diameter. The pole is then cut into 3/4 inch lengths, and a hole is made at either end with a toothpick. This is then set on the handle of a needle that has already been inserted into the body. The moxa is lit, and allowed to burn all the way down. Three such pieces are burned per needle. Before setting the moxa on the handle of the needle, a cotton ball is slipped down the handle of the needle, to rest on the patient's skin. Then a heavy piece of paper or cardboard is slipped down the handle to rest on the cotton ball. This will protect the skin from falling moxa ash. This method is good for patients with pain deep in the joints, for stiff shoulders and knees and tumors in the belly.

3.4.7 Indirect Moxa with Moxa Pole

In China today, moxa poles may be purchased ready-made in two formats. The "God's Needle" (or *Nim Ying*) moxa pole combines a number of herbs, in addition to the moxa, in a single pole. The pole is lit and, when well ignited, covered with 7-10 pieces of red cotton material. This shielded end of the pole is then applied to the acupuncture point until the skin appears pink-scarlet. It is helpful to have two such poles burning simultaneously, alternately re-lighting them as each begins to cool. Use additional pieces of cloth if the patient complains of the heat, replacing the cloth when it begins to char. When treating a number of points, switch between them as the point being treated becomes too hot for the patient.

The God's Needle is effective in the treatment of diseases involving numbness, hemiplegic conditions, and facial paralysis.

The second commonly used moxa pole contains moxa only. After it is lit, its burning end is raised and lowered above the skin, at a minimum distance of 1 inch from the skin's surface. Although this method is quite effective, it is difficult to apply without causing a blister. The pure moxa pole is especially effective in the treatment of itchy skin disease and ringworm.

It is also possible to apply the burning moxa pole around the handle of an inserted needle, and is an effective substitute for burning moxa directly on the needle handle, especially when many needles must be heated. The needle will transmit the heat to the point, and thus to the inside of the body.

Chapter Four
The Acupuncture and Moxibustion Treatment

4.1 *The Correct Time for Therapy*

According to the *Nei Ching*, one should not treat a patient with acupuncture in the following circumstances:

- On the day of the patient's first sexual experience
- After the patient has been drinking alcohol
- After the patient has been working very hard
- After a full meal
- If the patient is very hungry or thirsty
- After a long journey or after walking several miles
- If the patient is excessively frightened

Advise the patient to refrain from sex and alcohol after their first acupuncture treatment. After any acupuncture treatment, patients should not work extremely hard or eat a full meal. If a patient is frightened, they should rest for some time, and treatment should not proceed until his or her breathing becomes normal. After a long journey, or after walking several miles, the patient should rest for 1/2 to 1 hour before being treated with acupuncture.

4.2 *The Order of Points to be Stimulated*

In ancient times, acupuncturists treated head points first, and then body points; points on the front of the body, and then points on the back. For convenience, modern acupuncturists usually treat the arm first, then the leg, then the back, and finally the front of the body.

Treat the principal point first, and then the assistant points. For patients who are afraid of needles, and for light ailments, the assistant points may not be necessary.

For cases that require the treatment of painful points, treat the points that are not painful first, the painful points last. If the painful points are treated first, the patient might refuse to continue with the treatment; if the points that are not painful are treated first, the patient will be relatively more at ease when you do treat the painful points.

Treat points farthest from the painful area first, and gradually add points closer to the painful area. For example, for a severe headache, first treat the hand (LI-4) and arm (LU-7) to reduce the headache, then go on to treat the neck, (GB-20 perhaps), and finally the local head points.

For cases requiring the treatment of a large number of points, treat the body by areas, needling and applying moxa in one area first, then moving to the next area, until all points have been treated.

4.3 *Length of Treatment and Number of Points Required*

For light ailments, stimulate fewer points; for chronic and severe cases, more points should be stimulated. An acute toothache, for example, might only require the stimulation of LI-4. A chronic toothache or decayed teeth, on the other hand, would require the selection of additional points. In the treatment of madness, all 13 Ghost Points might be called for. A case of apoplexy might require the stimulation of all 12 Well points on the fingers.

If the patient's body is healthy, more points can be stimulated, and the stimulus applied for a longer period of time. Weak and nervous patients often cannot accept prolonged acupuncture needling without fainting, or feeling very weak. For these patients, often a single stimulation of the nerve with the needle is adequate.

In general, middle-aged men are capable of withstanding more needles and greater stimulus than women and small children.

Always pay attention to the patient's condition during treatment and inquire frequently about how he or she is feeling. If the patient reports feeling tired or dizzy, stop the treatment at once.

For patients with severe, painful problems, stimulate the points for longer periods of time by leaving the needles in the points; this will prevent the pain from returning.

There are many different theories about the number of needles that should be used and the length of time that should be spent in treatment. Many acupuncturists err by using a single method for all cases. Some use 30-50 needles in every case, seeming to imagine that if they use a lot of needles, a few would have to touch the right points. This is like using a machine gun to shoot a single person. Others use only 1-3 needles, regardless of the case's severity. These acupuncturists seem to think that the insertion of one needle will stimulate a miracle of sorts, and justify this method by pointing out that the old books contain acupuncture prescriptions involving only 2-4 points. However, in ancient times, people ate simpler food, lived healthier lives, and kept better hours, and as a result were more easily cured of acquired diseases.

Good acupuncturists should therefore understand that it is possible to use either too few or too many acupuncture points in a treatment. They must judge both the number of needles to be used, as well as the stimulation to be applied, for each patient and for each disease on a case-by-case basis.

4.4 *Determining the Length and Schedule of Treatment*

The following maxims should be helpful when determining treatment schedules.

• Acupuncture is not as effective when patients are treated only once a week because there will be no continuous, residual effect; pain will likely return in such situations. Many chronic cases will not recover with only one or two treatments, and may require as many as twenty to thirty.

• If the case being treated is a painful condition, and after the treatment the pain stops and then returns, you can treat the patient again that same day. If the first treatment does not make the patient tired, you can treat them once every day. If the patient feels tired after the first treatment, then you should wait two to three days before treating again.

• Patients who feel electric or strong sensations from the needle have a better prognosis than those in whom the stimulus is weak or difficult to obtain.

• Patients who experience a lot of relief after the first treatment usually recover more quickly than patients who feel no relief after the first treatment.

• New cases are easier to treat than old cases.

• Acute cases usually recover more quickly than chronic cases.

• Bodies that are basically healthy and strong are easier to cure than bodies that are weak.

• Patients with the ability to withstand strong needle stimulation and the pain from direct moxa usually recover more quickly than those patients with no patience for these procedures.

It is difficult to predict precisely how many treatments a patient might require for recovery. If you tell the patient that his or her case is easily treated, he or she will be happy indeed. However, if recovery does not occur as quickly as predicted, disappointment is inevitable. On the other hand, if you tell the patient that his or her case is difficult to treat and will take a long time, discouragement may prevent them from returning. Thus, it is usually best just to advise the patient whether or not the problem can be helped by acupuncture, and, if it can, simply to assure them that you will try your best.

4.5 *Observations During Treatment*

While treating, always pay attention to the following:

• Watch the patient's facial color and eye expression.

• Be certain that the patient has felt the stimulus by questioning him or her while needling. Unless the stimulus has been felt, your work will have been in vain.

• After 3-4 needles, ask the patient how he or she feels. If the patient is tired or upset, stop the treatment for several minutes before resuming.

• A patient's reaction to a first acupuncture treatment may be delayed for 10 to 30 minutes after the treatment. So that you can observe them, and monitor their reaction, ask the patient to wait for 10 to 30 minutes before leaving.

4.6 *Dealing with Commonly Encountered Problems During Treatment*

4.6.1 Swelling, Bleeding, and/or Pain Caused by Acupuncture Needles

If a vein is hit while inserting a needle, the point will bleed. If the needle completely pierces the vein, there will also be some swelling. If this occurs, lightly press and rub a cotton ball on the point. If the bleeding still does not stop, place a tiny piece of moxa (green bean size) on the point. When the swelling has been reduced, apply indirect moxa for a few minutes.

If the needle hits a tendon, there will be pain. In this case, and whenever a point feels painful, sore, or tired after needle application, use indirect moxa with ginger or the moxa instrument for 2-3 minutes on the point.

If a patient has an electrical sensation when the point is touched on the day following a treatment, lightly stimulate the same point with a needle, and follow with indirect moxa. The electrical sensation should disappear.

After using the needle in points near joints, the patient may feel some tightness and/or pain in the joint. Apply indirect moxa to these areas.

4.6.2 Difficulty Removing a Needle

When a needle is inserted too fast or too deep, the muscle will cramp up and bind the needle, making removal difficult. In this case, release the needle, and with your fingernail strike the muscle within a 4 to 5 inch radius of the point for 3-5 minutes. If the muscle does not cramp again, the needle should be easy to remove. Alternatively, insert a second needle about 1/4 inch from the first needle; this will also relax the muscle and make removal easier.

Some needles have small nicks or imperfections that might catch on muscle tissue when the needle is inserted and twisted, making removal difficult. Twist the needle in the opposite direction to release the tissue from the needle.

A needle can bend if a patient moves while the needle is still inserted. In this case, tell the patient to relax and return to their original position; then draw out the needle in the direction of the handle of the needle.

4.6.3 Broken Needles

With constant use, and due to the daily procedures of high-heat sterilization and cleaning with alcohol, all needles lose their elasticity and become brittle, increasing the risk of breakage during treatment. For this reason, ordinary steel needles that are used almost daily can only be used safely for three months; stainless steel needles used under the same conditions can be used for six months. If the body of the needle is damaged, or has had a history of being seriously bent and restraightened, it is much more likely to break. Finally, most needle breakages occur during deep insertion; always be careful during such procedures.

The combination of a poor quality needle and an unexpected movement of the patient during treatment is the most common cause for broken needles. A sudden cough, a quick and unexpected movement as a reaction to the needle stimulus, or a muscle cramp resulting from an insertion that was too rapid, might cause the sudden strain on the needle that will result in a break.

If the needle breaks without the patient's knowledge, it will be safer to attempt to extract it without telling them first. A patient agitated by such a situation might move in such a way as to drive the broken needle deeper into the body. If the patient is watching when the needle breaks, warn him or her not to move. During this time, the acupuncturist should remain as calm as possible. If the needle breaks at the point between the handle and the body, and the needle is still visible, use a pair of pliers to remove it. If there are no pliers, use forceps, tweezers, or even a pair of scissors. If the needle breaks in such a way that the tip is at the same level as the surface of the skin, press your fingers on the skin adjacent to the needle so that it protrudes from the skin's surface; then remove it with pliers, forceps, or tweezers. If the needle is below the surface of the skin, cut the skin with a sterilized knife, push down on the adjacent skin, and retract the needle. If the needle is broken deep within the muscle, it will have to be removed surgically.

4.6.4 Measures to Take When the Patient Faints

Patients with anemia of the brain, weak nerves, great hunger, and who experience exhaustion after hard work should be treated while lying down. These patients may experience lowered blood pressure, dizziness, nausea, blurred vision, sweating, enlarged pupils, a drop in body temperature, cold limbs, a weak heartbeat, and a weak or nonexistent pulse during the acupuncture treatment. When these symptoms do occur in such patients, the following procedures may help alleviate the problem:

• Remove all the needles and let the patient lie on the table for several minutes. The patient will soon return to a normal state.

• Use your fingernail to stimulate GV-26, LU-11, and PC-9.

• Needle GV-26 and ST-36.

• Give the patient some brandy to increase the circulation and to stimulate the heart.

• Apply moxa to GV-20.

• Give the patient smelling salts.

• After the patient revives, have them drink some hot water to increase their circulation.

To prevent a patient from getting dizzy during a treatment, the following procedures will prove helpful:

• Before treating, apply moxa (direct or indirect with ginger) on GV-20 to help raise the blood pressure.

• Have the patient chew a piece of ginger. The spicy taste will stimulate the upper palate, which will help strengthen the brain temporarily.

4.6.5 Treatment of an Infected Moxa Burn

After direct moxa, the patient may accidentally scratch the scar, causing it to become infected. There will be a little inflammation, or a little pus at the site of the scar. Clean the scar with hot water and carbolic acid, or water with lysol or Chinese tea. Dry it and apply Merchurochrome. By the next day it should have dried and formed a good scab. If the scar is deep, after cleaning apply pure moxa up to the level of the surface of the skin, and cover with a band-aid for several days; after this period of time the burn should be fairly well healed.

4.6.6 Treatment of an Inflamed Moxa Scar

The old book says that to be most effective, moxa should be applied until pus comes out of the burn. Although this is true in certain cases, especially in severe and chronic conditions, this method is not well received due to its severity. Indeed, application of direct moxa without stimulating pus secretion has been very effective for a number of my patients. Apply egg white several times a day after the hard scab drops off the scar to expedite the healing process.

4.6.7 Liniments and Ointments

Red Jade Ointment	
Step One	Measure 1 ounce of Boric Acid into a small jar.
Step Two	Slowly drop Mercurochrome into the Boric Acid until the Boric Acid has absorbed a sufficient amount to become slightly pasty (not too wet, not too dry).
Step Three	Add to the Mercurochrome-Boric Acid mixture 1 ounce of Vaseline, and mix well.

Red Jade Ointment is effective in the treatment of any open sores or ulcerations, as well as treatment of moxa burn ulcers. Put some ointment on a cotton ball, and apply to the ulcer until it has healed, changing the dressing once a day.

White Ointment	
Step One	In a small clay or stainless steel pot, put 1/2 ounce of Zinc Oxide, 1/7 ounce of Iodoform, 2 drops of Carbolic Acid (liquid), and 4 ounces of Vaseline.
Step Two	Boil gently while stirring until all the ingredients have melted and been combined.
Step Three	Pour the mixture through a filter, and store in a tightly closed jar.

Use **White Ointment** in the same manner as **Red Jade Ointment**, as well as for abscesses and carbuncles.

4.7 *Improving Your Skill as an Acupuncturist*

The needle is tiny, and the nerve invisible to the eye; acupuncture is precise and meticulous work. If your own body is not healthy, if you are tired, and lacking enough strength or spirit, you cannot properly treat your patients, and therefore cannot be an acupuncturist. If you are determined to be an acupuncturist, you should keep your body healthy and your spirit sufficient. Unhealthy habits should be stopped, and healthy habits cultivated.

If there are cases that you do not understand and cannot seem to help, you should search for understanding and solutions. Read other acupuncture books and journals to supplement your knowledge, and don't be ashamed to ask your teacher, experienced schoolmates, and acupuncture co-workers for advice. If you do this, your knowledge will increase, your fame will spread, and your patients will benefit greatly.

Never think that what you have learned is sufficient. Medicine is an ongoing knowledge, and, like a deep mine, your digging will never completely exhaust it. If you follow your teacher, and treat patients successfully, but later see books with different techniques, you must be able to distinguish between what you can successfully incorporate, and what contradicts your own successful experiences as an acupuncturist.

Chapter Five
Special Treatment Techniques

5.1 *Selecting the Points According to the Hours*

Before the use of the clock, the Chinese divided the day and night into 12 double hours, and assigned a name to each.

The Chinese Clock		
Time	**Chinese Name**	**Meridian**
11 PM to 1 AM	*Tzu*	Gallbladder
1 AM to 3 AM	*Ch'ou*	Liver
3 AM to 5 AM	*Yin*	Lung
5 AM to 7 AM	*Mao*	Large Intestine
7 AM to 9 AM	*Chen*	Stomach
9 AM to 11 AM	*Szu*	Spleen
11 AM to 1 PM	*Wu*	Heart
1 PM to 3 PM	*Wei*	Small Intestine
3 PM to 5 PM	*Shen*	Bladder
5 PM to 7 PM	*Yu*	Kidney
7 PM to 9 PM	*Shu*	Pericardium
9 PM to 11 PM	*Hai*	Triple Warmer

According to Chinese medical texts, *Chi* will completely fill a specific meridian at a specific hour. This phenomenon may be utilized in the treatment of disease. For example, headaches that occur regularly at 7 AM may be associated with the stomach meridian. By inserting a prismatic needle at the last point on the stomach meridian, ST-45, and squeezing out the dark blood until fresh, red blood appears, such morning headaches will be cured.

5.2 *Balancing the Sympathetic Nerves*

Many diseases are due to an imbalance between the left and right sympathetic nerves of the back. Each of these nerves controls the function of a specific internal organ, and, by this organ association, is related to one of the major meridians. Since all the major meridians, except for the Governing Vessel on the back and the Conception Vessel on the front, exist as bilateral pairs, we may treat such right-left sympathetic nerve imbalance by balancing the right and left sides of the related meridians. This method should be used when other methods prove ineffective.

To determine which pair of nerves are in a state of imbalance, a small heating instrument is used to measure the sensitivity of each right and left pair of meridian points on the ends of the fingers and toes. These measurements are then compared.

Using a stop watch, or a watch with a second hand, time the application of heat to the point at which the patient reports pain. The meridian that measures the longest application of the heating instrument before pain is reported is considered to be weak. To balance the sympathetic nerves, moxa is applied to the weak side, and a needle inserted into the strong side of the back *Shu* points related to the meridian that was tested.

To illustrate this procedure, coughing, which is usually related to a disorder of the lungs, may be tested to see if there is some sympathetic nerve imbalance associated with it. Using a small heating instrument on LU-11 (the last point of the Lung meridian at the end of the thumb near the nail), time the application of heat until the patient reports pain. If the left thumb feels the pain due to heat after 30 seconds while the right side takes 15 seconds, this indicates that the sympathetic nerve at the left lung is weak.

To treat this imbalance, needle BL-13 (the lung *Shu* point on the back) on the right (strong) side one time. Then apply 3 direct moxa (half rice grain size) to the left (weak) BL-13. After this treatment, the coughing will stop.

There are occasions when coughing is not due to a disorder of the Lungs. In these cases, it will be necessary to test all the meridian end points to determine the source of the imbalance.

This method of balancing the sympathetic nerves was invented by the Japanese acupuncturist, Mr. Chi-Yu Shi.

Balancing the Sympathetic Nerves		
Organ / Meridian to be Tested	**Test Point**	**Treatment Point**
Lung	LU-11	BL-13
Large Intestine	LI-1	BL-25
Pericardium	PC-9	BL-14
Diaphragm	Diaphragm Test Point†	BL-17
Triple Warmer	TW-1	BL-22
Heart	HT-9	BL-15
Small Intestine	SI-1	BL-27
Spleen	SP-1	BL-20
Liver	LV-1	BL-18
Stomach	ST-45	BL-21
8 Yu Meridians	On the third toe, outer corner of the nail	Between T-8 & T-9, lateral 1 1/2 finger divisions
Gallbladder	GB-44	BL-19
Bladder	BL-67	BL-28
Kidney	KI-1	BL-23

† At the lower, lateral corner of the finger nail of the middle finger

5.3 *Electric Needle Therapy*

A low-voltage D.C. electric generator, connected to the head of an inserted needle, will significantly reduce pain, sometimes offering complete relief within several minutes. This method is appropriate only for patients with a strong body, a healthy face, and a strong pulse; weak patients should be treated with direct or indirect moxa.

5.4 *Sha (Scratching) Therapy*

Although the Chinese word *Sha* literally means "sand," it has a wider, colloquial usage difficult to translate accurately into English. Its general meaning relates to the sandy texture of the skin in certain circumstances (sharks are called "sand-fish" in Chinese because of their skin texture).

The disorder we call *Sha* occurs as a result of abnormal and/or obstructed blood circulation in the joints or muscles. Often mistaken for rheumatism, *Sha* may produce such symptoms as tiredness and pain in the neck, back, arms, legs, and joints. If such *Sha*-induced pains or tired feelings in the muscles or joints are treated as though rheumatic in origin, only temporary relief may be expected, with symptoms reappearing after a few days.

To determine whether or not a person has *Sha*, forcefully press the painful area with the thumb. If the skin appears white and remains so for some time after the thumb is released, this indicates the presence of *Sha*.

To treat this condition, first use acupuncture at the painful area to lessen the pain. Then rub some oil or Vaseline onto the painful area, and scratch the skin with a smooth edged tool, such as the edge of a Chinese soup spoon. If *Sha* is present, red dots of *Sha* will appear at once. In severe cases, these dots may even be black. After these dots have appeared, the painful or tired feeling in that area will disappear at once. Instruct the patient to avoid starchy, fried, or roasted food for 24 hours after treatment; the *Sha* will not appear again.

5.5 *Bleeding the Fingertips*

In this method, a prismatic needle is inserted into the most distal points of the ten fingers until they bleed. Blood is pressed out until all the accumulated dark blood is removed, and fresh, red blood appears.

Although seldom used except in cases of extremely high fever, this method is often the only effective treatment of a condition of intense spasmodic abdominal pain called "twisting of the intestines." This condition occurs with *Sha*, and is treated by first bleeding the fingertip points and then scratching the abdomen to produce *Sha*.

Chapter Six
Ear Acupuncture

Ear therapy is especially effective in treating pain in the head, eyes, ears, nose, and throat. Each point of the outer ear is related to a specific part of the body (see the illustration below). By inserting needles into these areas, we may treat disease in the area of the body related to those points.

To make ear point location more precise, ear points may be pressed with a smooth probe to test for sensitivity. Alternatively, a metal ear probe may be connected to one electrode of a low voltage D.C. generator as the patient holds the other electrode. Touch the ear with the probe, and note the points that the patient reports as being painful. Insert needles into those painful points and allow them to remain there for at least 15 minutes. The disease will be cured and pain will disappear at once.

6.1 *Location and Effects of Acupuncture Points on the Ear*

6.1.1 Acupuncture Points on the Helix

1. Diaphragm: At the lower part of the crus of the helix. Used to help cramping of the diaphragm, skin disease, epistaxis, and uterine hemorrhaging.

2. Lower Segment of the Rectum: At the anterior portion of the helix at the same level as the **Large Intestine** point. Used in cases of dysentery, inflammation of the intestines, anal prolapse, fissures around the anus, piles, to help relax the anal sphincter, and to help relieve constipation.

3. Urethra: At the anterior portion of the helix at the same level as the **Urinary Bladder** point. For inflammation of the scrotum, genital itching, eruptions on the scrotum, and lumbar pain. For inflammation of the urethra and incontinence.

4. External Genital Organ: At the anterior part of the helix at the same level as the inferior crus of the antihelix.

5. Apex of the Auricle: At the upper part of the helix, facing toward the terminal portion of the superior crus of the antihelix.

6. Helix 1, 2, 3, 4, 5, & 6: At six equal intervals, beginning from the auricular tubercle of the helix and going downward to the middle of the lower margin of the auricular lobule.

6.1.2 Acupuncture Points on the Scapha

7. Fingers (digiti manus): At the scapha, above the level of the auricular tubercle. Used for finger sprain and inflammation of the fingernails.

8. Wrist (carpus): At the scapha, at the same level as the auricular tubercle. Used for sprained wrists and skin eruptions.

9. Shoulder: At the scapha, at the same level as the incisura anterior. Used for shoulder sprain and inflammation.

10. Elbow (cubitus): At the scapha, between the **Wrist** and **Shoulder** points.

11. Clavicle: At the scapha, at the same level as the **Neck** point. This point may be used in cases of inflammation of the shoulder joint, to treat a broken clavicle, and for pain in this area.

12. Shoulder Joint: At the scapha, between the **Shoulder** and **Clavicle** points.

6.1.3 Acupuncture Points on the Antihelix

13. Toes (digiti pedis): At the posterior part of the superior crus of the antihelix.

14. Ankle (malleolus): At the antero-superior part of the superior crus of the antihelix.

15. Knee (genus): At the superior crus of the antihelix, at the same level as the superior border of the inferior crus of the antihelix.

16. Ischium (os ischii): At the middle point of the superior border of the inferior crus of the antihelix, slightly toward the anterior side.

17. Buttock (natis): At the middle point of the superior border of the inferior crus of the antihelix, slightly toward the posterior side.

18. Abdomen: At the antihelix, at the same level as the lower border of the inferior crus of the antihelix. For cramps in the trunk region, to treat intestinal problems, disorders of the gallbladder, and urethral pain.

19. Thorax: At the antihelix, at the same level as the incisura anterior.

20. Neck (collum): At the notch between the borderline of the antihelix and antitragus.

21-23 Lumbo-Sacral Vertebrae, Thoracic Vertebrae & Cervical Vertebrae: A series of points lying along the curved rim of the cavum conchae on the antihelix. This line of acupuncture points could be separated into three segments if divided at the points **Lower Point of the Rectum** and **Shoulder Joint**. The upper segment belongs to the field of the lumbo-sacral vertebrae; the middle segment to the thoracic vertebrae; and the lower segment to the cervical vertebrae.

6.1.4 Acupuncture Points on the Tragus and the Antitragus

24. Ear (organon auditus): At the depression in front of the incisura anterior.

25. Nose (nasus): At the central point of the external surface of the tragus.

26. Pharynx and Larynx: At the inner surface of the tragus opposite to the orifice of the external auditory meatus. For inflammation of the pharynx and larynx, in cases of swollen uvula, and to treat dysphonia.

27. Internal Nose: At the inner surface of the tragus, slightly below the points **Pharynx** and **Larynx**. For any kind of nasal inflammation, epistaxis, and ulcers in the sinus membranes.

28. Apex of the Tragus: The upper projection of the tragus (at the upper rim of the projection if only one projection is found). Used to treat high fever and to reduce inflammation and pain.

29. Adrenal Gland (glandula supra-renalis): The lower projection of the tragus (at the lower rim of the projection if only one projection is found). This point adjusts body circulation, helps increase blood pressure, stops bleeding, reduces fever, stops inflammation, and is useful in cases of excessive sensitivity, skin disease, treatment of shock, rheumatism, and stimulation of the respiratory system.

30. Forehead (frons): At the antero-inferior portion of the antitragus. This point is used to treat chronic sinusitis, toothache, and dizziness.

31. Back of the Head (occiput): At the postero-superior part of the antitragus. Use this point for nervous system disorders, for disorders of the respiratory system, eye diseases, skin diseases, to reduce inflammation, to remove *Supp,* and for motion sickness.

32. *Ping Chuan:* At the apex of the antitragus. In the absence of a prominent antitragus, this may alternatively be located at the center point of the brim of the antitragus. Used to stimulate and control the respiratory system, and in cases of coughing, panting, and itching.

33. Subcortex: At the inner surface of the antitragus. Used to stimulate and to control the brain, to stop pain and inflammation, to calm the mind, for inflammation of the veins and arteries, in patients who show no palpable pulse, for gastroptosis, and in cases of uterine prolapse.

34. Internal Secretion: At the bottom part of the incisura intertragica. This point helps regulate all internal secretions, and may be used in cases of female disorders, problems involving childbirth, digestive disorders, rheumatism, and skin diseases.

35 & 36. Eye 1 & 2: At the inferior part of the incisura intertragica; **Eye 1** is in front, and used to treat cataract, dim vision, and any eye disease. **Eye 2** is behind. It is used for astigmatism, and in all eye diseases.

6.1.5 Acupuncture Points on the Triangular Fossa

37. *Shen Men:* At the bifurcation of the crus of the antihelix. This point controls the meninges, which in turn affects the brain's control over the body in general. Needling it can help comfort a painful situation, induce sleep, stop skin itching, and reduce inflammation.

38. Uterus: At the mid point of the anterior portion of the triangular fossa, just behind the anterior portion of the helix. Used for any female disorder, as well as male impotency and testicular inflammation.

39. Sympathetic: At the border line between the rim of the inferior crus of the antihelix and the curved brim of the anterior portion of the helix. This point effects the digestion, the respiratory system, the blood circulation, and the renal system. It controls the sympathetic and the autonomic nervous system.

6.1.6 Acupuncture Points on the Cavum Concha and Cymba Concha

40. Mouth (cavum oris): At the posterior wall of the orifice of the external auditory meatus. For ulcers in the mouth, inflammation of the tongue, and lockjaw.

41. Oesophagus: At the upper portion of the cavum concha, just below the crus of the helix.

42. Cardiac Orifice (ventriculus pars cardiaca): At the upper portion of the cavum concha and just below the crus of the helix, lying just behind **Oesophagus**.

43. Stomach (ventriculus gaster): At the upper portion of the cavum concha, just below the disappearance of the crus of the helix. Used for digestive disorders, diseases of the nervous system, and nervous breakdowns.

44. Small Intestine (intestinum tenue): At the lower portion of the cymba concha and above the crus of the helix. For poor digestion, intestinal gas, duodenal ulcers, and any disease of the heart.

45. Large Intestine (intestinum crassum): At the antero-inferior portion of the cymba concha, just above the crus of the helix. Used in cases of dysentery, intestinal inflammation, diarrhea, constipation, and piles.

46. Liver (hepar): Immediately posterior to the acupuncture point **Stomach** in the postero-inferior part of the cymba concha. Used for all eye diseases, blood diseases, rheumatic diseases, anemia due to iron deficiency, inflammation of the arteries and veins, and for patients with no palpable pulse.

47. Kidney (ren): In the upper part of the cymba concha, at the superior portion of the acupuncture point **Small Intestine.** Strengthens the entire body, used in cases of deafness, tinnitus, decreased hearing ability, eye disease, all female disorders, urinary problems, hair loss, to help stop the pain of broken bones, and in cases of loose teeth.

48. Urinary Bladder (vesica urinaria): At the antero-superior part of the cymba concha, just below the inferior crus of the antihelix. Used in cases of bladder inflammation, anuria, and bed-wetting.

49. Pancreas/Gallbladder (vesica fellea): At the posterior part of the cymba concha, just anterior to the points of the **Thoracic Vertebrae**. This point lies between **Liver** and **Kidney**. On the left ear, this point represents the pancreas, and may be used in cases of pancreatic inflammation, diabetes, and poor digestion. On the right ear, it corresponds to the gallbladder, and is used to treat inflammation of the gallbladder, gallbladder stones, tapeworms, and for all eye diseases.

50. Spleen (lien): The lower half of the **Liver** point on the left ear. For digestive disorders, withering of the muscles, piles with anal prolapse, and hemorrhaging.

51. Heart (cor): At the center of the deepest portion of the cavum concha. Use to strengthen the heart, to prevent shocks to a weak heart, to increase blood pressure, for excessive dreaming, insomnia, and inflammation of the tongue, larynx, and pharynx.

52. Lung (pulmon): On the circumference of the point **Heart**. Use for any problem of the respiratory system, for skin disease, hair loss, and inflammation of the sinus.

53. *San Jiao:* In the cavum concha, among the points **Internal Nose, Lung,** and **Internal Secretion.** Use this point in cases of diseases of the trunk, for the membranes that support the intestines, to affect the peritoneum and to treat urinary disorders. Use of this point will increase the platelet count. Combine with the point **Internal Secretion** for cases of dropsy.

6.1.7 Acupuncture Points on the Auricular Lobe

54. Vertex, Chin (mentum), Cheeks (buccae), Upper Jaw (maxilla), and Lower Jaw (mandible) are all located on the lobe, and should be located by probing for sensitivity.

55. Eye (oculus): At the central portion of the auricular lobule. Use in cases of unclear vision.

6.1.8 Acupuncture Points on the Back of the Ear

56. Depressing Groove: A curved vertical groove on the back of the ear.

57. Upper Back: At the cartilaginous eminence.

58. Lower Back: At the cartilaginous eminence.

6.2 *Ear Acupuncture Point Prescriptions*

General Ear Acupuncture Prescriptions		
Clinical Effect	**Primary Points**	**Secondary Points**
To calm the patient and induce sleep	*Shen Men* Kidney Forehead Occiput	Heart Subcortex
To comfort pain	*Shen Men* Apex of the Tragus Occiput Subcortex Sympathetic . . . as well as points corresponding to the diseased organ system	External Genital
To alleviate fear	Subcortex Heart Liver *Shen Men*	Gallbladder Spleen Kidney Occiput
To stimulate the brain	Heart Subcortex Sympathetic Adrenal Gland	Liver
To stop bleeding	Spleen Diaphragm Adrenal Gland	Heart Sympathetic
Diuretic points to relieve dropsy	Kidney Bladder *San Jiao* Spleen	Heart Lung

General Ear Acupuncture Prescriptions		
Clinical Effect	**Primary Points**	**Secondary Points**
To relieve muscle cramps	Sympathetic *Shen Men* Points relating to the specific meridian/organ	*Ping Chuan* Adrenal
To desensitize (in conditions of allergies, skin sensitivities, etc.)	*Shen Men* Internal Secretion Adrenal Subcortex	*Ping Chuan* Lung Large Intestine
To stop inflammation	Occiput Internal Secretion Adrenal Subcortex	Apex of the Tragus
To treat malaria	Internal Secretion Adrenal Subcortex	
To reduce fever	Subcortex Large Intestine Apex of the Tragus Adrenal Liver	*Shen Men* Adrenal (draw blood)
For night sweating	Heart *Shen Men* Internal Secretion Occiput	Subcortex Sympathetic Kidney
To alleviate dizziness	Forehead Kidney *Shen Men*	Occiput Liver

General Ear Acupuncture Prescriptions		
Clinical Effect	**Primary Points**	**Secondary Points**
To alleviate itching	*Shen Men* Internal Secretion Adrenal Related organ and meridian points	Occiput Lung Lumbar Vertebrae
To help clarify vision	Liver Eye Kidney Occiput	Eyes One & Two
To treat muteness	Heart Subcortex Mouth	*Shen Men* Kidneys Tongue
To balance the sympathetic and autonomic nerves	Sympathetic Subcortex Testicle Ovary	Kidney External Genital
To protect the liver	Liver Gallbladder Spleen Stomach	Testicle
To increase blood sugar	Sympathetic Adrenal Kidney	Subcortex
To decrease blood sugar	Pancreas Internal Secretion	Liver *Shen Men*
To decrease blood cholesterol	Liver *San Jiao* Small Intestine	
To expel poison	Liver Kidney Adrenal *San Jiao*	

Gastro-Intestinal Disorders	
Disorder	**Ear Points**
Gastric pain **Borborygmi** **Flatulence**	Abdomen Large Intestine Small Intestine Sympathetic Occiput Adrenal Subcortex *San Jiao*
Appendicitis **(acute and chronic)**	Vermiform Appendix Sympathetic Abdomen Large Intestine *San Jiao*
Cramping of **the diaphragm**	Diaphragm *Shen Men* Sympathetic
Inflammation of **the gallbladder** **Gallbladder stones** **Gallbladder pain**	Gallbladder Pancreas Liver *Shen Men*
Food Poisoning	Stomach Small Intestine Large Intestine Adrenal Internal Secretion Forehead Abdomen
To stop diarrhea	*Shen Men* Small Intestine Spleen Lung Sympathetic Kidney

Gastro-Intestinal Disorders	
Disorder	**Ear Points**
To alleviate constipation	*San Jiao* Large Intestine Subcortex Lower segment of the Rectum
To control excess acidity	Sympathetic Internal Secretion *Shen Men* Subcortex Liver Apex of the Tragus
To aid digestion	Stomach Spleen Right-ear Kidney Small Intestine *San Jiao* Pancreas Gallbladder Occiput
Indigestion and flatulence	Stomach Liver Spleen Large Intestine Small Intestine Subcortex Sympathetic
Acute or chronic inflammation of the stomach	Spleen Stomach Sympathetic Large Intestine Small Intestine Pancreas Gallbladder

Gastro-Intestinal Disorders	
Disorder	**Ear Points**
Gastric or Duodenal Ulcer	Stomach Duodenum Sympathetic Abdomen *Shen Men* Subcortex
Nervous Stomach	Stomach Duodenum Sympathetic Liver *Shen Men*
To stop vomiting	*Shen Men* Sympathetic Occiput Stomach
Gastroptosis	Stomach Spleen Subcortex Sympathetic Pancreas Gallbladder
Inflammation, Tuberculosis, or cramping of the intestines.	Large Intestine Small Intestine Sympathetic *Shen Men* Occiput
Acute Inflammation of the stomach and the intestines (vomiting and diarrhea)	Stomach Large Intestine Small Intestine Cardiac Orifice Diaphragm

Respiratory Disorders	
Disorder	**Ear Points**
Coughing **Panting** **Bronchitis**	*Ping Chuan* Lungs Adrenal *Shen Men* Occiput Spleen
Melancholia in the chest, **Chest pain**	Lung Thorax Heart Sympathetic
Influenza	Nasus Internus Pharynx Larynx Trachea Forehead
To stop coughing	*Shen Men* Lungs Adrenal Internal Secretion Pharynx Larynx Occiput
To treat cramping of the diaphragm	Diaphragm Liver Occiput Subcortex *Shen Men*
To stop panting	*Shen Men* Adrenal Lungs Kidney Occiput *Ping Chuan*

Circulatory System Disorders	
Disorder	**Ear Points**
Heart palpitations	Heart Small Intestine *Shen Men*
Arrhythmia	Heart *Shen Men* Subcortex Sympathetic Small Intestine
No palpable pulse	Subcortex Heart Adrenal Liver Spleen *Shen Men*
Hypertension	*Shen Men* Depressing Groove Heart Hypertension Subcortex
To stimulate the heart	Heart Subcortex Small Intestine Sympathetic Adrenal Gland Lung

Circulatory System Disorders	
Disorder	**Ear Points**
To treat irregular heart beat	Heart Subcortex *Shen Men* Sympathetic Small Intestine Lung
To raise the blood pressure	Heart Subcortex Lung Adrenal Gland
To lower the blood pressure	*Shen Men* Depressing Groove Hypertension Heart Subcortex Apex of the Tragus Sympathetic Bleed the veins at the back of the auricle
To increase blood volume	Heart Spleen Kidney Stomach

Urinary and Reproductive System Disorders	
Disorder	**Ear Points**
Impotency **Inflammation of the testicles** **Wet dreams**	External Genital Testis Internal Secretion Subcortex *Shen Men*
Acute and chronic kidney and bladder inflammation	Kidney Bladder Adrenal Sympathetic *Shen Men* *San Jiao*
Stones in the urinary tract	Urethra Kidney Sympathetic Subcortex
Anuria	Bladder Urethra Sympathetic External Genital
Bed wetting **Polyuria**	Kidney Bladder Subcortex Internal Secretion Subcortex *Shen Men* Encephalon Bed wetting point (between *Ping Chuan* and Encephalon)
To control excessive urination	Internal Secretion Subcortex *Shen Men* Kidney Sympathetic

Eye, Ear, Nose, and Throat Disorders	
Disorder	**Ear Points**
Menier's disease **Motion sickness**	Internal Nose Subcortex *Shen Men* Occiput Forehead
Any ear disorder	Internal Ear External Ear *Shen Men* Kidney Internal Secretion Occiput
To increase hearing ability	Kidney Ears Temples
Acute deafness	Encephalon Brain Stem Subcortex

Eye, Ear, Nose, and Throat Disorders	
Disorder	**Ear Points**
Any eye disorder	Eyes (3) Liver
Any nose disorder	External Nose Internal Nose Adrenal Internal Secretion For sinusitis, add Forehead
Pharyngitis **Laryngitis**	Pharynx Larynx Tonsils (4) Internal Secretion For chronic cases add Heart and *Shen Men*
Toothache	Tooth Extraction Anesthetic Points (2) Mandible Maxillary Mouth Cheek

Female Disorders and Problems with Childbirth	
Disorder	**Ear Points**
Menstrual pain	Uterus Sympathetic Internal Secretion Subcortex *Shen Men*
Irregular Menses **Uterine hemorrhage**	Abdomen Ovary Internal Secretion Encephalon Adrenal
Inflammation at the pelvic girdle **Leucorrhea**	Abdomen Internal Secretion Uterus Ovary Lower Segment of the Rectum Cavum Pelvis
Metritis	Uterus Internal Secretion Ovary Adrenal
Vaginal inflammation and itching	External Genital (2) Urethra Internal Secretion

Female Disorders and Problems with Childbirth	
Disorder	**Ear Points**
Pain following labor when the uterus is shrinking	Uterus Sympathetic Subcortex *Shen Men*
Uterine prolapse	Uterus Subcortex Internal Secretion
To increase lactation	Internal Secretion Spleen Kidney Mammary Heart Stomach
To assist in childbirth	Uterus Abdomen Subcortex Lumbar Vertebrae
To treat irregular menses	Uterus Ovary Kidney Internal Secretion

Disorders of the Nervous System	
Disorder	**Ear Points**
Bell's Palsy	Cheek Mandible Forehead Subcortex
Intercostal neuralgia	Thorax *Shen Men* Occiput
Neuralgia of the upper jaw	Maxillary Mandible
Trigeminal neuralgia	Maxillary Mandible Cheek
Sciatica	Nervus Ischiadicus Buttock *Shen Men*
Neuralgia of the neck	Neck Shoulder Joint Brain Stem
Sequelae of meningitis	Subcortex *Shen Men* Brain Stem

Disorders of the Nervous System	
Disorder	**Ear Points**
Neurasthenia **Excessive dreaming**	Subcortex *Shen Men* Occiput Kidney Heart Forehead
Headache **Dizziness** **Migraines**	Subcortex Occiput Vertix Forehead Temples *Shen Men*
Epilepsy	Spleen Stomach *Shen Men* Liver Forehead Heart Occiput Subcortex

External Disorders	
Disorder	**Ear Points**
Pain (from injury, post-surgical, joint)	*Shen Men* Subcortex Adrenal
Tendonitis and rheumatism	Sympathetic Spleen Points related to the painful area
Lumbago **Leg pain**	Lumbar Vertebrae Coccyx Nervus Ischiadicus Kidney Bladder
Headache following a spinal block	Lumbar Vertebrae Occiput Forehead
Piles, anal carbuncles and anal prolapse	Lower Segment of the Rectum External Genital *Shen Men*
Stiff neck	Clavicle Neck Cervical Vertebrae Occiput Internal Secretion
Skin disease	Internal Secretion Lungs Points related to the affected area

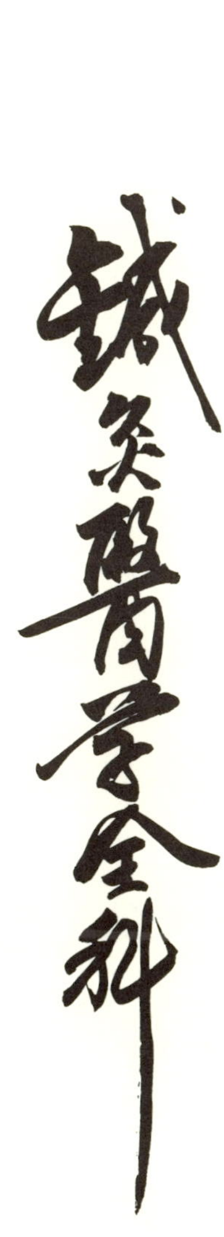

II

Traditional Chinese Diagnosis

Chapter One Looking

Diagnosis is the art of recognizing a disease by its cause, location, and symptoms. Although in Western medicine there are many different diagnostic techniques, in Chinese medicine there are only four: *looking, listening, asking,* and *taking the pulse.*

1.1 *Looking at the Face*

All illness is reflected in the face. Since each area of the face corresponds to a specific internal organ, by careful observation of the face during the course of any illness, the location and origin of a disease may be ascertained.

1.1.1 Parts of the Face and Related Organs

The forehead and the inner and outer corners of the eyes correspond to the heart. The heart corresponds to fire and to the color red. The tongue is the sprout (bud) of the heart.

The nose and eyelids correspond to the spleen. The spleen corresponds to earth and to the color yellow. The mouth is the opening of the spleen.

The left side of the face and both irises correspond to the liver. The liver corresponds to wood and to the color green. The eyes are the opening of the liver.

The right side of the face and the white part of the eyes correspond to the lungs. The lungs correspond to metal and to the color white. The nostrils are the opening of the lungs.

Both the cheek bones and the pupils correspond to the kidney. The kidney belongs to water and to the color black. The ears are the opening of the kidney.

1.1.2 Facial Color

A person suffering from the beginning stages of flu will have a gloomy face, lacking in normal shine. One who has been sick for a long time, and whose face suddenly becomes shiny and bright has a fairly serious condition. A dark face is also indicative of a serious condition.

In any case of long duration, a little yellow color on the face is not serious. This yellow color corresponds to the spleen and the stomach, and shows that the spleen and stomach are still alive, and that the patient will be able to maintain his or her appetite. An appetite will prevent a serious disease entity from causing death. Patients with a long history of disease, without some yellow color on the face, and with white, red, green, or blue coloring are difficult to cure.

1.2 *Looking at the Eyes*

The eyes are the spirit of the five solid organs, and are the essence of the water of the kidney. The pupil corresponds to the kidney. If there is enough water in the kidney, the eyes will be clear; if heat has injured the kidney, or if the kidney itself is overheating, the eyes will be unclear and dim. The old book says that there are two essential qualities to the kidney — fire and water. If a patient's eyes are clear, this indicates either that the disease has not gone deep inside the body, or that the body is overcooling. If the eye is red or yellow, the disease is deep within the body.

A person who is suffering from a severe disease, but who still likes to open his or her eyes to see visitors, has a yang condition, a condition that is not yet critical. A patient who keeps his or her eyes closed, and does not look at any one is suffering from a yin condition, which is quite dangerous. If a patient feels that the eyelids are very heavy, this indicates that the nose will soon start to bleed.

Yellow eyeballs indicate a jaundiced condition. In some conditions, the patient's eyes will stare upward, to the side, or straight ahead, with the eyes wide open and round, or suddenly recessed. This indicates the death of one or more of the five solid organs.

Sudden blindness from one eye after a long and chronic illness indicates a lack of *chi*. Sudden dimness in both eyes indicates a lack of blood circulation. Both these conditions are dangerous.

1.3 *Looking at the Nose*

The nose corresponds to the spleen. If the nose is a little blue, this indicates that the patient is suffering from gastric pain. If the nose is a little dark, this indicates that there is much phlegm inside of the body. If the nose is a little yellow, there is *Supp* and overheating in the body; if it is white, there is a lack of *chi* in the body. If the nose is red, there is overheating in the lungs. If the nose is a shiny, natural skin color, this indicates that the body is healthy.

A stuffed and/or runny nose indicates coldness in the lungs. A flu with dry nostrils indicates that there is an overheating condition of the muscles of the body, and that nose bleeding will probably follow. If the patient looks like he or she is going to sneeze, but can't sneeze, this indicates that the body is overcooling and has caught cold. A stuffed nose with thick mucus means the patient has caught cold (wind) and that the body is overheating. Snoring indicates rheumatism in the body.

When the nostril is dry and black, like a chimney, the body has ''yang poison'' and deep overheating; this is a very dangerous sign. A cold sensation upon exhalation from the nostril, with dark, wet nostrils, indicates ''yin poison'' and deep overcooling. If the wings of the nose move while breathing, the lungs are in critical condition, (e.g., pneumonia). After labor, if a woman's nostrils become dark or bleed, her stomach and lungs are dying.

1.4 *Looking at the Mouth*

The lips are the principal of the muscles and the spirit of the spleen. By looking at the color of the lips one can determine whether or not the patient's disease is deep or superficial. If the lips are dry and parched, this indicates an overheating condition of the muscles of the body. Lips that are parched and black indicate a dangerous situation; parched and red lips are not as serious.

If the lips and mouth are red and swollen, this indicates that there is deep overheating in the muscles of the body; if the lips and mouth are blue or dark, this indicates that there is deep overcooling in the muscles of the entire body.

A bitter taste in the mouth indicates overheating in the gallbladder. A sweet taste in the mouth indicates overheating in the spleen. Injury caused by eating too much will result in uncomfortable feelings in the stomach and abdomen, and loss of taste while eating.

Dryness in the mouth and throat indicates overheating in the kidney. A patient with difficulty talking probably has a history of muscle cramping or apoplexy.

In general, the prognosis is poor for patients who have been ill for a long time, and who show the following symptoms and signs:

- Cramping in the tongue and the lips
- Up-turning and cyanosis in the lips
- Trembling of the lips
- Evidence of a dark ring around the mouth
- Mouth breathing which favors exhalation
- Cramping of the mouth in the shape of a fish's open mouth

1.5 *Looking at the Tongue*

The tongue in general is the sprout of the heart. The tip of the tongue indicates the condition of the heart organ. Behind the area of the heart is the area corresponding to the lungs. The center of the tongue corresponds to the spleen and stomach. Both sides of the tongue correspond to the liver and gallbladder. The root (rear) of the tongue corresponds to the kidney.

1.5.1 Internal-External, Overheating-Overcooling

An absence of tongue coating in a patient suffering from the flu with a high fever indicates that the disease is external, and has not yet penetrated inside the body.

A fresh, red-colored tongue indicates an overheating condition. When dryness accompanies redness, this indicates a deeper overheating condition. Conditions such as cramping of the tongue and "double tongue" also indicate deep overheating conditions.

A moist tongue, which is also shallow pink or pale, indicates an overcooling condition.

1.5.2 Tongue Coatings and Meridian Relationships

A white coated tongue indicates that a flu has penetrated half way into the body, and has affected the gallbladder meridian. A yellow coated tongue indicates that the flu has fully penetrated the body's interior. A purple tongue indicates that the sickness has penetrated into the pericardium meridian. A black tongue indicates that the disease has entered both the heart and the kidney meridians.

1.5.3 Tongue Papillae

A pink tongue with small papillae indicates that the body is healthy. A tongue whose papillae have disappeared, and whose surface is as smooth as the outside of the kidney, is called a "mirror tongue." The presence of such a tongue indicates that the patient will die.

1.5.4 Tongue Coatings, Colors and Organ Relationships

A tongue with a thin white coating in a mouth which isn't dry, indicates that the disease is still on the outside of the body. A tongue covered by a dull white powder-like coating indicates that the lungs are dying. A white, granular coating on the tongue, which gradually thickens, indicates that the flu has entered the stomach, and is gradually changing to "fire" (overheating). When the thick coating changes to a yellow color, this indicates that the "fire" condition has established itself, and that there is deep overheating and *Supp.* If this condition is not alleviated, the coating will become black, and the overheating will have become quite severe.

A dark coating on the tongue indicates a dangerous condition. Occasionally, such a case will stop deteriorating. In a case where the black coating is initially like small shells or scales, which eventually drop off, and the whole tongue becomes bright red and dry, the body lacks liquid and has excess fire.

Several of the above cases are dangerous, indicating that the disease has penetrated deep inside the body.

If the spleen and stomach are overcooling, the muscle of the tongue is pale and excessively wet, with no coating, and the patient's lips are pale and the face whithered, this indicates that the patient has diarrhea or overcooling *Supp*, and that there is no fire in the spleen. If the tongue has a very thin yellow coating, this indicates that the spleen is starting to overheat. If this yellow coating is thick, the stomach is overheating and has *Supp.* If this thick yellow coating gets cracked and dry, it indicates a strong overheating condition of the stomach.

A very red tongue tip, often with a thorn-like surface, indicates that there is overheating in the heart. If the tip is thick and black, with a dry coating, often with a thorn-like surface, this indicates that there is deep and strong overheating throughout the body.

If the teeth and lips are dry and dark, this indicates that the stomach has been injured. If there is a thin, dark, and wet coating on the tongue, this indicates that cold has gotten inside of the body and has directly entered the stomach. It also indicates that the patient has an overcooling condition in the kidney. If the whole tongue is purple, without a coating, this indicates that the body is overcooling, with a little fever. In another condition, a patient who has recovered from a disease and has a purple and shiny color on the tongue, or dryness in the throat, and who does not like to drink cold liquids, is manifesting indications that the kidney is without water.

Conditions such as cramping of the tongue and double tongue indicate extreme overheating. Stiffness of the tongue, shortness, hardness, unconsciousness with a dry tongue, or difficulty speaking clearly, all can be indicative of dangerous conditions.

1.6 *Looking at External Symptoms*

Conditions of overcooling are indicated by:

- shortness of breath
- general body weakness
- pale face and lips
- diarrhea
- shortness of micturition
- stiffness and coldness of the four limbs

Conditions of overheating are indicated by:

- rough breathing
- delirium
- an inability to lie calmly (constant tossing and turning)
- constipation
- deep yellow or red-colored urine

1.7 *Signs of Death*

- When the body smells very bad, the muscles have died.
- When the tongue and the scrotum cramp up, the liver has died.
- When the mouth cannot close, the spleen has died.
- When the muscles of the body become swollen and both lips turn out, the stomach has died.
- When the hair becomes straight and all the teeth become dry, the kidneys have died.
- When all the hair of the body becomes dry as though burnt, the lungs have died.
- When the face becomes dark and the eyes are fixed straight ahead, or are half-closed and blind, the yin has died.
- When the eyes sink in and the muscles above the eyes become slack and the perspiration does not flow, but comes out like pearls or glue, the yang has died.
- When the patient spreads the arms out like Christ crucified, or with eyes fixed looking up, the Great Yang (small intestine and bladder meridians) has died.
- After the disease is gone, when panting and diarrhea continue, the spleen and lungs have died.
- If the eyes look straight ahead and the eyelids cramp into circles recovery is unlikely.
- If the patient has saliva with bubbles coming from the mouth, and a red or blue and dark face; blue and swollen lips so that the philtrum depression disappears; hair and eyebrows go straight up; all the nails become dark; the palm becomes smooth, without creases; the umbilicus depression disappears; the top of the foot swells; the patient's moans sound like

snoring; the pulse sinks down without a root; the face becomes blue and the pulse disappears, the eyes are blind; and sweat becomes like oil, these signs indicate that the liver is dead.

• When the muscles of the eyebrows become slack, the gallbladder has died.

• When all the fingernails fall off, and the patient can't stop shouting and scolding, the nerves have died.

• If the patient has to move the shoulders to breathe, and the head is turned looking backward, the heart will die very soon.

• If all the hair goes straight up and can't be bent and the patient never stops sweating, the small intestine has died, and death will come in six days.

• If the mouth is cold, the feet swollen, the belly feels very hot and swells up, and the patient has constant diarrhea, then the lungs have died, and death will come in five days.

• If the patient has pain on the spine, the body becomes very heavy and he or she cannot turn to the side, the stomach has died, and death will come in five days.

• If the ear becomes dry and withered, the tongue swollen, and there is blood in the urine and feces, the muscles have died, and death will come in nine days.

• If the patient's mouth is always open, with more air going out than coming in, the lungs have died, and death will come in two days.

• If the patient has diarrhea many times a day, the large intestine has died.

• When the teeth dry up, the feces are black, the eyes yellow, the patient has severe lumbar pain, and excessive perspiration, the kidneys have died.

Chapter Two
Listening

Listen to the patient's voice. A low voice indicates that the body is weak (empty). A loud voice indicates that the body is strong (full).

If the patient's speech is such that when he or she starts talking it is loud and heavy, but then becomes weaker and lower, this indicates that a flu has penetrated deep within the body. A patient who initially talks very slowly and lazily and then becomes louder and more energetic in his or her speech, is suffering from injured *chi.*

Listen to the patient's cough. A loud cough indicates that the patient has sufficient *chi.* A weak, difficult cough indicates that the patient lacks *chi.*

Delirium indicates strong overheating, probably accompanied by dry feces in the intestines. The delirious patient will start talking coherently but will soon trail off into nonsense. This patient's spirit will be troubled, and personal awareness diminished. Hiccoughing, or phlegm sounds from the throat while breathing, are both bad signs in conditions of delirium. When a patient's voice starts changing, it means the soul has started to depart.

An angry, shouting patient has a diseased liver. A patient that laughs a lot has a diseased heart. A patient who is always thinking, and occasionally singing, has a diseased spleen. A very worried, often crying patient has diseased lungs. A patient who groans a lot and is often frightened has a diseased kidney. A patient with dyspnea, short, rough, quick, and loud breathing has strong overheating of the body. A patient whose breathing is short, weak, and accompanied by small wheezing sounds, is "empty" and has weak *chi.*

Hiccoughs at the beginning of an illness can be from either an overheating or an overcooling condition. Hiccoughs that appear after a patient has been sick for a long time indicate that the stomach is dying. If a patient's voice doesn't change during illness, this is a good indication that the condition is not critical; if the voice *does* change, and speech becomes nonsensical, the condition has become critical.

Chapter Three
Asking

When qucstioning a patient about his or her condition, the practitioner should focus upon twelve areas of inquiry: *sensations of heat and coolness; perspiration flow; sensations in the head; patterns of urination and bowel movement; eating and drinking habits; sensations in the epigastrium; sensations in the hypogastrium; aural acuity; sensations of thirst; medical history; causative factors of the presenting illness;* and *menstrual patterns.* Information gathered from the patient about his or her own perception of the problem, especially with respect to these areas of inquiry, will allow the acupuncturist to structure a clear diagnosis, and to establish a more effective treatment plan.

3.1 *Ask About Hot and Cold*

The quality of cold is yin, the quality of heat is yang. Ask the patient how cold or hot he or she feels to determine if he or she is more yin or yang. If the patient has the flu, he or she will feel cold even though they have a high fever, and there will be no way to make him or her warm.

If overheating *causes* the flu, the patient will have intermittent fevers and chills. If overheating *precedes* the flu, the patient will feel warm when covered with a blanket. If the disease process starts with a headache, high temperature, and cold sensations, it is the flu. If the disease process starts with a stomachache and diarrhea, the flu is combined with overeating.

3.2 *Ask About the Perspiration Flow*

If the patient has the flu, ask if there has been perspiration. If there has been no perspiration, the disease is more superficial. If there is flu and perspiration with a high fever, the flu is more internal, and is accompanied by overheating.

3.3 *Ask About Sensations in the Head*

A case of the flu, compounded by a headache, indicates that the flu is serious. A case of the flu without a headache indicates that the condition is not critical because the patient's body is weak. If the patient feels dizzy at the beginning of the flu, the dizziness was caused by either wind, fire or phlegm. A patient who feels dizzy after an attack of the flu has a weak body and lacks *chi.* You can look at the patient's body to help determine from which meridian the disease began.

Sensations of heaviness throughout the body accompanied by difficulty moving indicates a serious problem. If the body feels light and easy to move, this indicates that the case is not so severe. If the patient has a lot of *Supp,* rheumatism, or an overcooling condition, the body will feel heavy and painful even in the absence of fever.

Symptoms of a deep yin condition include: a heaviness throughout the entire body; stiffness and coldness in the four limbs; a desire to sleep in the fetal position (with the knees pulled up); cold sensations in the absence of fever; a desire to keep the eyes closed; photophobia; and a desire to avoid seeing people.

Symptoms of ''yin poison'' include generalized body ache (as if one has been beaten up); profound heaviness, and difficulty moving. If the body is overheating, the circulation is good and the body is light. If the body is overcooling, the circulation will be poor and the body heavy and painful.

When the body is cramped, either the arms and legs will be cramped, or the whole body will cramp backwards into a curve. If the patient's head is heavy, and tends to drop forward, this indicates that the *chi* (nerves) of the spine has been damaged. A head that won't stop shaking, hair that stands straight like it's been well combed, and a head raised up are dangerous signs. A patient with a long-term illness who touches the edges of his clothes and/or searches everywhere on top of the bed, or tries to catch invisible nothings from the air, has lost their spirit and their soul is in trouble.

A patient who has been sick for a long period of time, but whose skin is still shiny, is not in such a critical condition. However, if the skin is dry and without shine, the condition is critical. A patient whose large muscles have completely wasted away cannot be helped.

3.4 *Ask About the Urine and Feces*

If the patient has dysuria, or if the urine is deep yellow or red, this indicates that the patient is overheating. If the urine is clear, this indicates overcooling. If the urine is white like rice wash water, overheating *Supp* is centering in the lower half of the body.

A patient with constipation is "full" overheating. A patient with long periods of diarrhea or dysentery is "empty" and weak. If the feces are mixed with white or clear liquid, the patient is overcooling. If the feces are deep yellow or red, the patient is overheating.

3.5 *Ask About Eating and Drinking*

In general, for any disease, if the patient retains their appetite, the condition is not critical. A patient with no appetite has a serious problem. A possible exception to this rule is the patient who has gotten sick from overeating; they will lose their appetite without being in a particularly dangerous situation.

If the patient likes sweet tastes, this indicates a weakness of the spleen. If the patient likes sour-tasting foods, the liver is empty.

3.6 *Ask about the Chest and the Upper Abdomen (Epigastrium)*

If the chest feels full and painful, the disease has come from the stomach and has reacted upwards. If the chest isn't painful, but the area under the chest becomes swollen, this is an indication of the accumulation of gas. If the patient has panting first and the chest becomes swollen, the disease is from the lungs. If the chest is full before panting starts, the disease is from the spleen. A patient who is thirsty, but vomits after drinking liquids, has stagnant liquid in the stomach.

Certain signs on the epigastrium will help determine if the disease is internal or external. Using your hand, lightly press the upper abdomen; if the disease is still located on the body's surface, or if is has penetrated only halfway into the body, entering the gallbladder meridian, the abdomen may be neither swollen nor painful. A disease that has completely penetrated the body's interior will cause the abdomen to be swollen and painful. If the swelling and pain are persistent, this is an indication that the disease has spread throughout the entire body. In China, one would prescribe herbs to move the bowels in order to help this case. If the abdominal swelling decreases following treatment, and the pain continues but has lessened, the disease, though internal, has not yet spread throughout the entire body. If the patient catches cold and feels a lot of pain in the upper abdomen, and the pulse sinks and slows, this indicates that the body is overcooling and that the flu has penetrated. This kind of patient needs warming herbs.

3.7 *Ask About the Lower Abdomen (Hypogastrium)*

Using your hand, press lightly on the lower abdomen. If the lower abdomen doesn't feel hard and painful to the touch, the disease is not deep inside the body. If the disease is deep within the body, the lower abdomen will be hard and painful to touch. If the patient's urine is normal but the feces are black, the patient is hemorrhaging internally. If the lower abdomen is painful up to the umbilicus and hard to the touch, and the patient has frequent, short urination, this indicates the presence of dry feces in the large intestine (constipation). If the lower abdomen is swollen and the feces are normal, the patient is suffering from bladder congestion and anuria.

3.8 *Ask if the Patient has Experienced Hearing Loss*

After the flu and a high fever, if a patient becomes deaf, the problem is very severe.

3.9 *Ask About the Patient's Thirst*

Thirst during a flu can be caused by either overheating or overcooling. If the patient likes to drink cold water, he or she is probably overheating. If the patient likes to drink hot water, he or she is probably overcooling. If the taste in the mouth is bitter, the patient is probably overheating. If the taste in the mouth is salty, the patient is probably overcooling. An insipid or sweet taste in the mouth indicates that the spleen is overheating. If overeating preceded the flu, there will probably be a sour taste in the mouth.

If the patient is thirsty but is not able to drink, he or she is probably overcooling. If the patient's mouth feels hot, and he or she drinks a lot of water, there is probably overheating. If the patient is very thirsty, and is delirious and has constipation, this indicates strong, ''full'' overheating. A patient who constantly drinks little sips of water, with normal feces and urine, has an overcooling ''empty'' body.

3.10 *Ask About the Patient's Medical History*

Ask for the patient's medical history to determine if and how the present case relates to past problems.

3.11 *Ask What Precipitated the Problem*

Find out how the condition started to help determine how to treat it.

3.12 *Ask About the Menstrual Cycle*

Female problems are often connected with menstrual patterns. Ask if menstruation has been delayed, irregular, nonexistent, or excessive, or if the patient has been pregnant, to help determine the patient's problem.

Chapter Four
Taking the Pulse

4.1 *Locating the Pulse*

The pulse is located at the three positions on the wrist that correspond to the three wrist points LU-7, LU-8 and LU-9, located at the inner edge of the radial bone. The middle position, LU-8, called the "bar," is used as a guide in accurately locating the proper pulse positions. The bar pulse is found at the eminence of the radial styloid bone, and is felt with the middle finger.

Distal to the bar pulse is the "inch" pulse, located at LU-9, the point behind the metacarpal bone. The inch pulse is felt with the first finger.

The third position, the "foot" pulse, is located on LU-7. It is felt with the ring finger.

The pulse is felt at three depths at these three positions: on the skin's surface (called *floating*), at a middle depth (called *medium*), and near the radial bone (called *sinking*). Using one finger at a time to palpate each position, sometimes you can find only one position that is abnormal.

In general, each pulse position corresponds to a yin-yang pair of organs or meridians. On the left hand the first position (inch) is used to diagnose the condition of the yin-yang pair, heart-small intestine, as well as the pericardium. The second position (bar) on the left hand is used to diagnose the condition of the yin-yang pair, liver-gallbladder. The third position (foot) on the left hand is used to diagnose the yin-yang pair, kidney-bladder, as well as the small intestine. In addition, the three positions of the left hand are used to diagnose the blood, because the heart is the master of the blood, and the liver is the storeroom of the blood.

On the right hand, the first position (inch) is used to diagnose the condition of the yin-yang pair lung-large intestine, as well as the chest area in general. The second position (bar) on the right hand is used to diagnose the yin-yang pair spleen-stomach. The third position on the right hand is used to diagnose the kidney (*Meng Men*)-triple warmer, and large intestine. The kidney (*Meng Men*) is a yin organ; the triple warmer and large intestine are yang organs. The old book says that the left side corresponds to the kidney, the right side to the is the Life Door (*Meng Men*), and that the root of the triple warmer starts at the Life Door. The three positions of the pulse on the right hand are used to diagnose the condition of the *chi*. The spleen and stomach receive and digest food; the large intestine is involved in the process of elimination; the triple warmer regulates the body. All rely on the *chi*.

4.2 *An Outline of the Pulse*

To diagnose accurately by the pulse, it is necessary to understand the four basic characteristics used to describe the pulse when in the presence of illness: *floating, sinking, slow,* and *fast*. A healthy pulse is neither floating nor sinking, neither fast nor slow, with an average rate of 72 beats per minute.

4.2.1 The Floating Pulse

If the pulse feels strong when the surface of the skin is palpated, yet disappears upon deeper pressure, this pulse is said to be *floating*. The floating pulse is usually a sign of external disease, but can, in certain cases of emptiness, indicate internal disease as well.

4.2.2 The Sinking Pulse

The *sinking* pulse is not encountered until one presses nearly to the bone. Although the sinking pulse usually indicates internal disease, it occasionally occurs in certain kinds of external flu conditions.

4.2.3 The Slow Pulse

A pulse of less than sixty beats per minute is a *slow* pulse. A slow pulse diagnoses the yin of the body, and thus indicates a condition of overcooling and weakness. The slow pulse can be floating or sinking. A slow, floating pulse indicates that there is overcooling *on* the body. A slow, sinking pulse indicates that there is overcooling *inside* the body. The slow pulse usually is used to diagnose the solid organs, but is used occasionally to diagnose the hollow organs.

4.2.4 The Fast Pulse

A *fast* pulse beats more than 80 times per minute, and is used to diagnose the yang of the body. A pulse rate of 120-140 beats per minute indicates a critical condition, and that the yang is overheating. The fast pulse can be floating or sinking. The fast, floating pulse indicates that there is overheating on the surface of the body (as in a flu). The fast, sinking pulse indicates that there is overheating inside the body. The fast pulse is usually used to diagnose the yang and the hollow organs. But sometimes the solid organ diseases will also have a fast pulse, as in tuberculosis.

In summary, the floating pulse relates to the yang and to external conditions, and accompanies wind (cold or flu) and emptiness (weakness). The sinking pulse is used to diagnose the yin and internal problems, and accompanies *Supp* and fullness. The slow pulse is used to diagnose disease in the solid organs, and accompanies overcooling. The fast pulse is used to diagnose the hollow organs, and accompanies overheating or dryness.

4.3 *The Eight Pulses as First Described by Chen Siu Yuen*

The four basic pulses described above (*floating, sinking, fast,* and *slow*) may now be further defined by describing additional pulse characteristics within those pulse types. Such refinements are another important aid to accurate pulse diagnosis.

4.3.1 The Floating Pulse

A strong floating pulse is a **great** pulse. The great pulse indicates overheating on the body.

A weak floating pulse is an **empty** pulse. An empty pulse indicates a lack of *chi.*

A very weak floating pulse is a **scattered** pulse. The scattered pulse indicates that the blood has decreased. This pulse is felt when pressed very lightly. If slight pressure is added, the pulse disappears; the empty pulse would not disappear under heavier pressure.

When the floating pulse feels like one is touching the stem of a green onion, it is called a **hollow** pulse. This pulse indicates that the patient has lost a large amount of blood. The hollow pulse is superficially floating and wide, and the middle part of this pulse is empty when pressed.

When the floating pulse feels like a drum it is called a **leather** pulse. This indicates more blood loss than the hollow pulse. This pulse has the feeling of the leather of a drum, superficially wide, hard, and hasty. Deeper pressure on this type of pulse yields no palpable pulse.

A floating pulse that is also gentle and narrow is a **soft** pulse, and is an indication of *Supp.* This pulse is palpable only superficially. It is thin, fine, and soft, like a piece of cotton floating on water.

4.3.2 The Sinking Pulse

A deeper sinking pulse, palpable only upon heavy pressure to the bone, is a **hidden** pulse. This pulse is beneath the muscle near the bone. The hidden pulse indicates that the flu is deep within the body. This pulse can sometimes be found only at one position, and is not necessarily found at all three. It also indicates that there may be just one organ that has been affected by the deep flu.

The **firm** pulse is a hard, sinking, leather pulse, and feels like the skin of a drum, though harder, and indicates excessive overcooling of internal organs, poor blood circulation, and poor functioning of the organs.

A narrow, soft, sinking pulse is a **weak** pulse, indicating that the patient has a lack of blood, and poor functioning of the internal organs. It is found in patients who have been sick for a long time.

4.3.3 The Slow Pulse

A **slowed-down** pulse beats at a rate of 60-65 beats per minute, and does not necessarily indicate illness.

A **rough** pulse indicates insufficient blood and weakly functioning organs. The movement of this pulse is rough, choppy, slow, and thin.

A slow pulse that irregularly stops and starts is a **knotted** pulse, and indicates an obstruction in the body from a chill, or an accumulation of undigested food and phlegm in the body.

A slow pulse that regularly, rhythmically stops and starts is an **intermittent** pulse. This pulse usually beats three, four, or five times for each stop. It indicates that one or two of the solid organs are dying, and that the patient will soon die.

4.3.4 The Fast Pulse

A fast pulse that feels smooth to the touch is a **smooth** pulse. According to the old book, this pulse feels like pearls rolling in a basin.

A healthy person with a smooth pulse has abundant blood. A woman with a smooth pulse at the six positions is probably pregnant. A patient with a smooth pulse is suffering a phlegmatic and/or overheating disease.

A fast pulse that feels as if it is turning to both sides is a **tight** pulse. A tight pulse is tight and strong, like a long piece of rope, fastened at one end, pulled tightly at the other, while being twisted back and forth from side to side. This pulse indicates overcooling, and the patient will in most cases be in pain and/or have body cramps.

A **hurried** pulse is a fast pulse qualified by irregular stops and starts, and indicates that the patient is suffering from a critical condition of deep overheating.

A fast pulse with one position that feels like it is moving up to touch the finger, like a shaking, rapidly moving, headless, tailess bean, is a **moving** pulse (usually found at the bar position). This pulse is indicative of internal hemorrhaging and/or a war between the body's yin and yang. It could also indicate a condition of overflowing yang, which would be accompanied by a high fever and profuse perspiration. It could also indicate a condition of overflowing yin, with the patient having a high temperature and insufficient fluids in the body.

If the floating pulse is fast it indicates external overheating.

4.3.5 The Fine Pulse

The narrow and thin pulse, which feels analogous to the silk threads of a spider's strand, is a **fine** pulse. It gives the sensation of being thin, straight and soft, and indicates empty organ functioning.

A difficult-to-find fine pulse is a **minute** pulse. This pulse denotes a dearth of blood and *chi,* and a lowered temperature — a critical condition. If a patient is suffering from an acute illness and has this pulse, it indicates a sudden, severe weakening of the patient's body, but still with hope of recovery. A patient suffering from a chronic condition who has the minute pulse may not be able to recover from his or her illness.

A fine pulse that is narrow, thin, and floating is an **immersed** pulse. The quality of this weakly beating pulse is that it is as narrow as a spider's thread, floating like a flower petal floats on water. This pulse denotes an exhausted bone marrow and deficient body fluids — a dangerous sign.

A sinking, powerless, fine pulse is a **weak** pulse. This pulse is similar to the hidden pulse but is very weak. It indicates a chronic lack of nourishment, yang, and *chi,* and very weak functioning of the organs. This pulse is often found on patients who have been sick for a long time.

4.3.6 The Big Pulse

The **big** pulse indicates yang and fullness in the body, the patient suffering from an overheating disease. A big pulse is two times as wide as the normal pulse.

An overflowing, big pulse is a **grand** pulse. This pulse feels full, large and overflowing, fully filling the three pulse positions, faltering in strength upon slight pressure. A grand pulse can indicate either deep overheating in the body or weakness from a long illness, loss of blood, or loss of body fluids due to diarrhea.

A wide, hard, big pulse is a **strong** pulse. This pulse feels strong under either light or hard pressure, and indicates a dormant, deep overheating. For a patient with an acute condition who has this pulse, the disease has developed very rapidly and extensively.

4.3.7 Short

A patient has a **short** pulse when the inch position and foot position are abbreviated on either end. This indicates that the body has been weak from birth. Great care should be taken when treating this patient with acupuncture or herbs.

4.3.8 The Long Pulse

The **long** pulse is palpable from LU-10 to LU-5. This indicates the patient has a super strong body by birth, a rare occurrence. A normally beating long pulse indicates that the person has good health. A fast, raging, long pulse indicates strong and deep overheating. A strong and long pulse is a **strong** pulse.

In the six conditions of external, internal, overcooling, overheating, empty, and full, if the pulse is short, the patient is weak from birth, and you should protect the patient's health when treating (i.e., don't use powerful medications and/or strong therapy on this patient). If, in one of the six conditions, the pulse is long, the body is strong by birth, or the patient has an overheating disease, you should use very powerful medications.

4.4 *Some Notable Exceptions of Pulse Types in the Diagnosis of Disease*

Floating pulses do not always indicate external disease. If the patient has a lack of blood in the body, and the pulse is floating and weak, it indicates internal disease. Although the sinking pulse indicates that there is internal disease, a patient in the early stages of a flu, who catches cold too often, with the hair follicles of the skin temporarily closing up, will have a pulse that will also be sinking and tight.

Although the slow pulse indicates overcooling, a patient who has recently recovered from the flu, with a slight temperature, will often have a slow and slippery or smooth pulse. The narrow pulse indicates that the body is "empty", but a patient with severe pain in the body will often have a narrow, sinking pulse. Although the big pulse indicates that the body is "full," a patient who has had a long period of sickness, and whose blood and *chi* are empty, will have a pulse that will be bigger than normal.

4.5 *Non-Pathological Variations of the Pulse*

In patients with thin bodies, the *chi* will be on the surface of the body, and therefore their pulse will be a little floating. In fat patients, the *chi* is inside the body and the pulse will sink slightly.

The impatient individual will normally have a rapid pulse, greater than 80 beats per minute. The individual with an unhurried, slow disposition will normally have a pulse beat of less than 60 beats per minute. Seventy beats per minute for this patient would indicate overheating.

For the patient with a long body, you should spread the fingers a little over the pulse positions to find them correctly; for the short patient, the fingers should be compressed together to touch the pulse correctly.

People who live in the north will have stronger pulses; southerners will have weaker pulses.

According to the old book, the pulse changes with the seasons. In the springtime, the pulse is somewhat like the string of a musical instrument; in the summertime the pulse is like a hook; in autumn the pulse is like a hair; in winter the pulse is like a stone.

A strong, young body will have a slightly bigger pulse. The old body will normally have a pulse that is a little empty. A baby's pulse should beat 100 times per minute.

After drinking a lot of wine, the pulse will beat much faster; after eating dinner, the pulse is bigger than usual; after walking a long distance, the pulse will be a little fast; after not eating for several days, the pulse will be empty; in big girls and women the foot pulse will be bigger than the inch pulse, the right hand pulse bigger than the left. A girl that is old enough to marry but abstains from sex, and does not marry, as well as nuns in convents, will have weak or immersed pulses.

4.6 *The Yin and Yang of the Pulse*

In front of the bar pulse is the yang pulse; behind the bar pulse is the yin pulse. The floating pulse is yang; the sinking pulse is yin. The fast pulse is yang; the slow pulse is yin. The strong pulse is yang; the weak pulse is yin. If the pulse is long and big it is yang; short and narrow it is yin. Therefore, if the pulse is floating, big, smooth, moving, or fast, it is yang. If it is sinking, weak, rough, string, or slow, it is yin.

Yin-Yang Aspects of the Pulse	
Yin	**Yang**
Foot Pulse	Inch Pulse
Sinking Pulse	Floating Pulse
Slow Pulse	Fast Pulse
Weak Pulse	Strong Pulse
Short & Narrow Pulse	Long & Big Pulse
Rough or String Pulse	Big or Smooth Pulse

The floating pulse indicates external disease; the sinking pulse indicates internal disease. Big or wide pulses indicate that the body is too strong. The weak pulse indicates that the body is empty. The smooth pulse indicates that the blood is excessive in the body. The rough pulse indicates a lack of *chi* in the body. The moving pulse shows excessive yang in the body; the string pulse shows excessive yin in the body. The fast pulse indicates that disease is in the hollow organs; a slow pulse indicates the disease is in the solid organs.

4.7 *Determining Potentially Fatal Conditions Through the Pulse*

If the pulse is strong and yang when the patient first starts getting sick, but after several days it starts changing into a weak, yang pulse, this indicates that the patient's yang is almost vanquished, and that death is imminent. If the yin pulse predominates when the patient first starts getting sick, but later it changes into the yang pulse, this indicates that the patient's yin is almost depleted, and that the patient will soon die, like the light of the candle which flames and sputters just before dying. A patient who has been sick for a long period of time, with no pulse at the inch and bar positions, but still with a pulse at the foot position, will still not die. If the patient's foot pulse is gone and only the inch and bar pulses are beating, it is like a tree with damaged roots and green leaves: still alive, but not for long.

Another way to diagnose death by the pulses is to press the pulses very hard until the beating is not distinguishable; then loosen your fingers. If the pulse returns quickly, it indicates that the patient will not die. If the return is delayed, the patient is dying.

The above diagnostic techniques are also related to the kidney pulses. The old book says that both foot pulses come from the kidneys; if the kidneys are dead, the above conditions of death will also exist. A patient who is excessively weak from a long period of illness should have an empty pulse: if the pulse is big, this indicates that the patient is dying. A patient who has the flu should have a yang pulse; if the pulse is yin the patient is in a critical condition.

4.8 *The Female Pulse*

A normal female pulse has the foot pulse bigger than the bar and the inch; the right hand pulse a little bigger than the left. If the foot pulse is small, rough, or smooth but the smoothness is irregular; or the left foot or bar pulse is sinking, these are indications of irregular menstruation. If the three parts of the pulse beat equally, and the patient is without sickness, and the menstrual cycle has stopped, the patient is pregnant. If the woman has a weak body, but the foot pulse is beating and is hard to press, the woman is pregnant. A woman whose menstruation has stopped who is also sick, with both pulses beating normally, is pregnant.

A young woman with a weak and rough foot pulse, an overcooling uterus, and fear of coldness, will have difficulty getting pregnant. A middle-aged woman with the above symptoms would not be able to conceive.

A Pregnant Woman's Pulse

If the foot pulse is smooth and active, or if the left-hand inch pulse moves strongly, it indicates that the woman is pregnant. If the pulse is smooth and fast and further pressure on the pulse makes it spread away on both sides of the fingers, the woman is three months pregnant. If the pulse is smooth, gentle, with regular intermittent beats (i.e, the pulse stops and starts, but always for the same number of beats), the woman is two months pregnant. If under hard pressure the pulse feels fast but does not spread under the fingers, it indicates that the woman is five months pregnant.

If the foot pulse is normal and active, the woman is pregnant. If the left foot pulse is big and active, the baby should be a boy. If the right inch pulse is big, it's a girl. If a pregnant woman is without indicative discrepancies in the inch position pulse, examine the foot pulse to determine the baby's sex. Just before labor the pulses should be normal. In ancient times, only 1 out of 10 women would survive who bled excessively after bearing their first child, and whose foot pulse became indistinguishable.

4.9 *The Child's Pulse*

If a child is under five years of age, you will not be able to diagnose the pulse as you would in an adult. Rather, the child's pointing finger (boy's left, girl's right) is used to diagnose the child's illness. In children who are ill, a vein will become visible under the outside edge of the first finger crease (the **Wind Gate**). If this vein is red or purple, the child is overheating. If the color is red and the skin outside of the vein is white, the child has the flu. If the line is blue, the child will have convulsions. A white vein line indicates chronic indigestion. A black line indicates that the child's condition is very critical.

If the vein is visible up to the second finger crease (the **Chi Gate**), this indicates that the problem is severe. If the vein is visible up to the third finger crease (the **Life Gate**), then the child is in danger. If the vein extends to the center of the palm, this indicates that the child is cold. If the vein runs down to the palm and then turns alongside of the hand, the child has an condition of chronic indigestion. A child's face and lip color are also good indications of his or her condition.

In children over five, use one finger to touch the whole pulse. A rate of 90-100 beats per minute is normal; over 100 beats per minute is overheating; under 90 beats is overcooling. If the baby is under one year, we can use the forehead to diagnose their condition. Touch the baby's forehead with the pointing finger lying along the hairline, the ring finger along the eyebrow, the middle in between. If the three fingers feel hot, the baby has caught a cold, and will probably have a stuffed nose and coughing. If the three fingers feel cold, the baby has the flu accompanied by overheating, a high fever, vomiting and diarrhea. If the upper two fingers feel hot, this indicates that the baby is overheating in the upper half of the body, overcooling in the lower half. If the ring and middle fingers are hot, the baby has been frightened by something. If only the pointing finger is hot, the baby has indigestion.

4.10 *The Seven Strange Pulses*

Do not treat patients who have one of the following seven pulses.

1. If a pulse feels like the erratic food-picking of a bird, picking and stopping, the liver has died.

2. If a pulse feels like a roof leaking, with long pauses between beats (drops), the stomach has died.

3. If the pulse feels like the residual vibrations of a strummed guitar string, the kidneys have died.

4. If the pulse feels like many tangled strings, the spleen has died.

5. When there is no foot pulse, only an inch pulse, and it's like a fish swimming with only the tail moving, the heart has died.

6. A shrimp-swimming pulse, a pulse which suddenly jumps and then becomes barely perceptible, indicates that the large intestine has died.

7. A thin, bubbly, boiling-water pulse, weak to the touch, disappearing under slight pressure, indicates that the lungs have died.

鍼灸醫學全科

III

Traditional Chinese Medical Theories

Chapter One
The Origins of Disease: The Six Evils

Chinese medical textbooks mention six causative factors as the origin of disease, the so-called "Six Evils." Although the actual translation of this phrase is "Six Lewdnesses," because of the potential for misunderstanding by English-speaking readers, I have chosen to substitute the word Evil for the word lewdness, as I have seen it translated in other English acupuncture books. These Evils are *Wind, Cold, Sunstroke, Supp, Dryness,* and *Fire*.

1.1 *Wind*

Wind in this sense does not refer to moving air or blowing wind, but to catching a cold or a flu.

1.2 *Cold*

Cold refers to the physiological condition of overcooling. In such conditions, a patient will have a lowered body temperature, low blood pressure, pale face and lips, and a general feeling of cold all over.

1.3 *Sunstroke*

This refers to the same condition understood by modern medicine as heatstroke or heat exhaustion.

1.4 *Supp*

Supp has been translated as "wetness" or "humidity." These are accurate, though limited translations of this condition. *Supp* is the Cantonese transliteration of the Chinese word 濕, pronounced *Shih* in Mandarin. Since there are over 15 words with the pronunciation *Shih* in Mandarin, I have chosen to render the Cantonese name for this fourth Evil.

Supp refers to a commonly found internal condition. When I was young, I was the disciple of Tsue Hong Ping, who taught me Chinese herbal medicine. It is through his explanation of *Supp* that I came to understand the origin and nature of this condition. It is that explanation that I offer here.

According to Dr. Tsue, *Supp* is the accumulation of undigested food on the walls of the stomach and the intestines. The symptoms include generalized body fatigue; tiredness in the four limbs; a wet coating on the tongue; loose and sticky bowel movement, which in some cases may change to diarrhea or dysentery, turbid urine, and poor appetite. If the *Supp* accompanies an overcooling condition, the tongue coating will be white. In the case of *Supp* with overheating, this coating will be yellow.

1.5 *Dryness*

Dryness refers to a physiological lack of body fluid. This condition results in a thickening of the blood, dry mouth and nose, parched lips, and thirst.

1.6 *Fire*

In a condition of fire, the patient's internal body temperature will be elevated, there will be high blood pressure, the entire body will feel hot to the touch, there will be great thirst, constipation, and deep yellow urine.

Chapter Two
The Theory of the Five Elements

In ancient times, physicians explained the interelationships among the five solid organs — heart, lungs, liver, spleen and kidneys — by using the *Law of the Five Elements.* According to this theory, each of the Five Elements —Fire, Metal, Wood, Earth, and Water— was associated with a specific organ: the heart with Fire; the lungs with Metal; the liver with Wood; the spleen with Earth; and the kidneys with Water. Thus, the observable forces of nature and the constant flow of mutual production and restraint among life's phenomena could be applied to an understanding of the body's physiological functions, and to the process of health and illness.

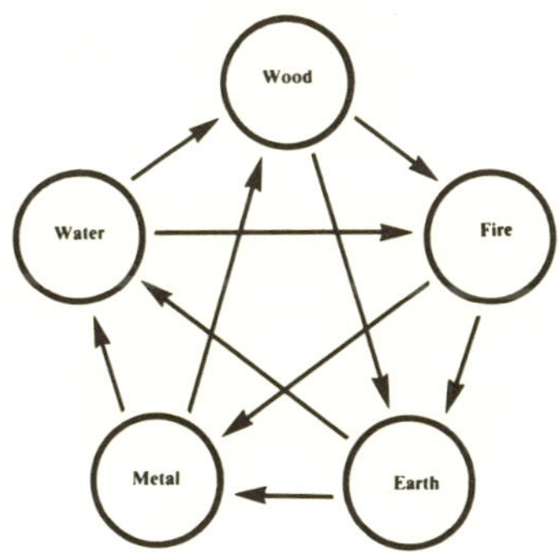

2.1 *The Production of the Five Elements*

Fire produces Earth: Life and growth on the earth are made possible by the fire of the sun. Anything burned by fire will produce some ash, and thus return it to the earth.

Earth produces Metal: Metals are mined from the earth.

Metal produces Water: In China, metal means gold; thus, where there is gold, there should also be a spring or water.

Water produces Wood: Wood needs water to sustain life and to grow.

Wood produces Fire: In the process of burning, wood is used for heat and warmth.

2.2 *Restraint of the Five Elements*

Fire restrains Metal: Metal, although hard, can be melted by Fire.

Metal restrains Wood: The metal ax or saw readily cuts wood.

Wood restrains Earth: Although earth is hard, it is penetrated by the roots of plants and trees, which can even break up rock.

Earth restrains Water: Earth dykes hold water during floods.

Water restrains Fire: Fire is quenched by water.

2.3 *Explanation of the Connections Between the Five Elements*

The old books obviously do not offer a modern, scientific explanation of the process by which the organs supply (produce) and control (restrain) each other. Perhaps the organs supply and control each other by certain of their internal secretions, which would effect the autonomic and sympathetic nerves that control and regulate them. However, until adequate research is completed which will add to our understanding of these phenomena, we can only speculate about their physiological basis.

Although Five Element Theory is not included in most classical medical books, we have found it to be true through observation of the organ functions themselves. For example, the heart corresponds to Fire, the liver (Wood) supplies power to the heart, and the kidneys (Water) control the power of the heart. Therefore, the heart is controlled by both the kidneys and the liver. If the liver is too strong, and the kidneys too weak, the liver would be supplying too much power to the heart, and the kidneys would not be able to control the power of the heart. The power of the heart will overflow, causing it to overheat and beat too fast.

Similarly, if the liver (Wood) is too weak, and unable to supply adequate power to the heart, the kidneys (Water) will be too strong, and exert too much control over the heart. The power of the heart will thus be weakened, and it will overcool and beat slowly.

If every organ is normal, the body is healthy: one diseased organ upsets the balance of all other organs.

Five Element Correspondences					
Element	**Fire**	**Metal**	**Wood**	**Earth**	**Water**
Organ	Heart	Lungs	Liver	Spleen	Kidneys
Color	Red	White	Green	Yellow	Black
Taste	Bitter	Spicy	Sour	Sweet	Salty
Sound	Laughter	Crying	Anger	Singing	Groaning
Master	Blood	Skin and Body Hair	Nerves	Muscle and Flesh	Bone
Beauty	Eye	Eyebrow	Nails	Lips	Hair
Opening	Tongue	Nose	Eyes	Mouth	Ear
Hidden Entity	Spirit	Strength	Soul	Ideas	Will
Tongue	Tip	Behind the Tip	Sides	Center	Back
Eye	Canthus	Sclera	Iris	Lids	Pupil
Pulses	Grand	Floating	String	Smooth	Sinking, Hard (Stone)

2.4 *The Five Colors*

The heart corresponds to Fire and to the color red. The lungs correspond to Metal and to the color white. The liver corresponds to Wood and to the color green. The Spleen corresponds to Earth and to the color yellow. The kidney corresponds to Water and to the color black.

A patient's facial color can reveal internal problems. Chinese herb books prescribe herbs by their color to aid the color-related organ. Colored foods or meats will aid color-related organs. Sometimes, however, the color of meats and herbs are not consistent with their function.

2.5 *The Five Tastes*

The bitter taste enters the heart; the spicy taste enters the lungs; the sour taste enters the liver; the sweet taste enters the spleen; the salty taste enters the kidneys.

Unless eaten in excess, the taste that enters an organ helps that organ. Since the liver controls the nerves, excess sour foods will over-strengthen the nerves and cause cramping. Since the muscles and the lips correspond to the spleen, the Earth element, and since the liver corresponds to Wood, which restrains Earth, excessive sour foods will also cause the muscles to wither and the lips to curl.

The skin and body hair correspond to the lungs. Since the lungs correspond to Metal, and the heart to Fire, and since Fire restrains Metal, excessive consumption of bitter-tasting foods will hurt the lungs, causing dry skin and loss of body hair.

The bones and head hair correspond to the kidneys. Since the kidneys correspond to Water, the spleen corresponds to Earth, and Earth restrains Water, excessive consumption of sweet-tasting foods will cause soreness of the joints and loss of head hair.

Since the nerves and fingernails correspond to the liver, the liver corresponds to Wood, the lungs correspond to Metal, and Metal restrains Wood, excessive consumption of spicy-tasting foods causes body cramping and withered fingernails.

Since the blood comes from the heart which corresponds to Fire, the kidneys belong to Water, and Water restrains Fire, too much salt hurts the blood causing a blood color change.

Our understanding of the function of the five tastes may be employed in the following maxims:

The sour taste enters the nerves. If the nerves are diseased, avoid sour-tasting foods to prevent the nerves from pain and cramping.

The bitter taste enters the bones. In any bone disease, avoid bitter-tasting foods or the four limbs will be difficult to raise.

The sweet taste enters the muscles. In any disease of the muscles, avoid sweet tasting foods to avoid the muscles becoming swollen.

The spicy taste enters the chi. In any *chi* disease, avoid spices or the *chi* will ‘‘spread-out’’ (decentralize) and become weak.

The salty taste enters the blood. Avoid salt if there is a blood disease, for excessive salt will thicken and cool the blood, and the patient will become very thirsty.

2.6 *The Five Masters*

The heart is the master of the blood, and blood circulation depends on the power of the heart. Abnormal blood is a reflection of heart problems.

The lungs are the master of the skin and body hair; a problem in these areas would be related to a problem with the lungs.

The spleen is the master of the muscles and flesh. Diseased muscles and flesh reflect a diseased spleen.

The liver is the master of the nerves, and diseased nerves reflect a diseased liver.

The kidney is the master of the bone. Diseased bone reflects a diseased kidney.

2.7 *The Five Openings*

The opening or sprout of the heart is the tongue. A diseased tongue reflects a diseased heart.

The nose is the opening of the lungs. Any nose problem reflects diseased lungs.

The eyes are the openings of the liver. Eye disease usually comes from a diseased liver.

The mouth (or lips) are the opening of the spleen, and problems with the mouth or lips reflect a diseased spleen.

The ear is the opening of the kidneys and its condition reflects the condition of the kidneys.

2.8 *The Five Hidden Entities of the Organs*

The spirit is hidden in the heart; thus the condition of a body's spirit relates to the condition of the heart. Strength is hidden in the lungs: with strong lungs, the patient will have strong *chi*. The soul is hidden in the liver. According to religious ministers, the soul relates to affections and sensations. Conceptions, ideas, thinking, and singing are hidden in the spleen. Inclination (the will) is hidden in the kidneys. Thus, a strong willed person should have strong functioning kidneys.

2.9 *Parts of the Tongue*

The tip of the tongue corresponds to the heart, the area behind the tip corresponds to the lungs, the central area corresponds to the spleen, both sides correspond to the liver, and the root of the tongue corresponds to the kidneys. Colors, and/or coatings on different parts of the tongue will supply information on related organs.

2.10 *Parts of the Eyes*

The eye as a whole corresponds to the liver. The red muscle at the inner canthus corresponds to the heart, the red muscle at the outer canthus belongs to the pericardium. The white part of the eyeball corresponds to the lungs, the upper eyelid to the spleen, the lower eyelid to the stomach, the iris to the liver, the pupil to the kidneys. If the eye becomes diseased, find which part was afflicted first to understand which organ is diseased.

2.11 *The Five Sounds*

The five sounds correspond to the five solid organs. Laughter corresponds to the heart; crying to the lungs; anger to the liver; thinking and singing to the spleen; groaning and fear to the kidneys. Listen to the predominant sounds the patient makes to understand which organ is diseased.

2.12 *The Five Sick Pulses*

With a diseased heart, the patient will have a grand pulse; with diseased lungs, a floating pulse; with a sick liver, a string pulse; with a sick spleen, a smooth pulse; with diseased kidneys, a sinking and hard (stone) pulse.

2.13 *The Five Dying Conditions*

When the heart is dying, the patient will raise the shoulders to help impaired breathing, and turn the head to look toward one side.

When the lungs are dying, the body hair will drop out as if it's been burned, and the patient will exhale more than inhale. The abdomen will become hot and swollen, and the patient will have constant diarrhea. When dying, the lungs are not able to supply life to the hair or to the breath. When the Yin organ dies, the complementary Yang organ, in this case the large intestine, also dies. When the large intestine deteriorates, such symptoms as diarrhea, hot sensations, and a swollen abdomen will result.

When the liver dies, there is cramping on the tongue and scrotum, and an oil-like perspiration over the entire body. The liver meridian circumscribes the sexual organs; death of the liver therefore causes cramping of the scrotum. The cramping of the tongue occurs because the liver cannot adequately supply power to the heart. With no Wood the Fire also dies. The oil-like sweating is a special symptom of the liver dying.

When the spleen dies, the patient's body starts smelling badly, and closing the mouth becomes difficult. The spleen controls the flesh and the mouth. When the spleen dies the flesh dies, giving off the rotten smell, and the mouth becomes immobile.

When the kidneys die, the hair on the head becomes straight, the teeth become dry, the diarrhea black, the eyes yellow, and the patient experiences severe lumbago and excessive sweating. The kidneys control the bones, the hair on the head is the spirit of the kidneys, and the teeth correspond to the bones. When the kidney dies, the patient's hair becomes straight and the teeth dry up. The color black corresponds to the kidneys, thus black diarrhea would indicate that the kidneys are dying. The eyes correspond to the liver, and the liver corresponds to Wood. The kidneys correspond to Water and supply power to the liver. With no Water, the Wood also dies. The kidneys have a connection to the lumbar area, and death of the kidneys causes pain here. The excessive perspiration is called "Losing Yang." When the sweating finishes, the patient will die.

2.14 *Treating Internal Disease by the Five Element Correspondences*

The *Mother and Son Law* is another important principle of Five Element Correspondence. In the production cycle of Five Element theory, the organ that produces energy is called the "mother." The organ that receives the energy is the "son." Thus, since Wood supplies power to Fire, the liver is considered the mother and the heart the son. The heart produces the power of the spleen; thus the heart is the mother, the spleen the son. The spleen supplies the power to the lungs; therefore the spleen is the mother and the lungs are the son. The lungs supply the kidneys; therefore, the lungs are the mother, the kidneys the son. The kidneys supply power to the liver; the kidney is then the mother, and the liver is the son. The old book says: "If the son is weak, stimulate the mother, if the mother is overheating, sedate the son." With herbs, one can easily use this principle to treat the patient, but with acupuncture, few people understand how to achieve this.

Since the heart is the mother of the spleen, if the heart is overheating and you want to sedate the son, this can be done by bleeding SP-1, thus drawing down the power of the spleen. This weakness of the spleen will stimulate the heart to supply more energy to the spleen to balance its weakness. The loss of power in the heart will reduce its overheating. This is how to "sedate the son when the mother is overheating." Fire is the son of Wood; the heart is the son of the liver.

Similarly, if the heart is weak, but the liver is not supplying strength to the heart, we can apply direct moxa to BL-18 (the liver yu) to strengthen the liver (mother), thereby supplying more power to the heart (son). This is the way to "stimulate the mother when the son is weak."

If an organ of the body is weak, we can use points on its meridian to help the patient. If this is not successful, then we can use the connection of the Five Elements.

2.15 *A Five Element Justification for Organ Transplant Failures*

Several years ago, heart and kidney transplants were attempted on various patients. Many patients with heart transplants lived for about one year after surgery; kidney transplants did not give the patient many more years of life. The patients' "new" hearts worked well, but they developed lung problems, such as bronchitis, and many died from pneumonia. Because the heart corresponds to Fire and the lungs to Metal, this means that the heart controls the power of the lungs. It would seem that the new heart cannot control the power of the lungs. The spleen still supplies power to the lungs, and the lungs get stronger and stronger until they develop an overheating condition. One day the patient catches cold or the flu, and pneumonia results. Because the lungs are strong and overheating, the pneumonia will get worse and worse. The ''new'' heart cannot control the lungs, the penicillin is unable to cure the pneumonia, and the patient dies.

A patient with a kidney transplant often develops liver problems. The kidneys correspond to Water, and the liver to Wood. The Wood, without Water, will dry up and die. When the original kidney is removed, and there is no more connection with the liver, no more power to the liver, the liver will also wither up and die, and the patient will become jaundiced and then die. This is a proof of the Five Elements connection.

Chapter Three
The Theories of Yin—Yang and Chi

3.1 *The Theory of Yin and Yang*

According to the old book, good health depends upon the harmonious interaction of the body's Yin and Yang. If one element is in excess, the body will be sick. Chinese medicine seeks to balance the body's Yin and Yang. The whole world can be classified as either Yin or Yang. The sky is Yang, the Earth is Yin. The sun is Yang, the moon is Yin. Daytime is Yang, nighttime is Yin. Fire is Yang, Water is Yin. Man is Yang, woman is Yin. The left side of the body is Yang, the right side is Yin. The back of the body is Yang, the front is Yin. Outside the body is Yang, inside the body is Yin. "Full" is Yang, "empty" is Yin. Hot is Yang, cold is Yin.

If the body or the world had only the Yin quality, nothing would live; if only Yang, nothing would grow.

3.2 *The Theory of Chi*

Any movement of the air can be termed *chi.* The air gun is the *chi* gun. The air window is the *chi* window. Atmospheric pressure is *chi* pressure. Breathing is *chi* breathing. Windpipe is pipe of *chi;* smelling is smelling of *chi.* Air bladder is *chi* bladder. Air balloon is *chi* balloon. Air breathing out is *chi* exhaling. Air breathing in is *chi* inhaling. Oxygen is life *chi.* Air pump is *chi* pump. Color of the face is *chi* color. Strength of muscle is *chi* strength.

The Chinese classics refer to two systems in the body: the blood system and the *chi* system (breathing, belching, flatulating). People who talk loudly have enough *chi.* People who can run for a long time have enough *chi.* People who can talk a long time have long *chi.*

When the needle is inserted into a point and the patient feels the stimulation, we say that the patient has "gotten the *chi.*" Since the "nervous system" per se was unknown in ancient times, the word *chi* was used to refer what we know now to be the actions of the nerves. However, the nervous system alone cannot explain the phenomenon of needle stimulation. In many instances, the direction of the stimulus does not follow the anatomical pathway of the nerves. For example, although insertion of the needle in LI-4 does indeed stimulate a nerve, the powerful effect that this point has on the face and jaw cannot be explained by the "nervous system" of Western medicine. The concept of *chi,* then, is both subtle and complex, and has not yet been fully explained by modern science.

Chapter Four
Diet Therapy

Chinese doctors always counsel their patients about diet and sex, and a good doctor understands the role that diet plays in a patient's illness. Unsuitable foods and drinks, consumed when ill, can make the patient's condition worse, and possibly hasten death. Almost all Western medical doctors often ignore the vital aspect of nutrition, and thereby often prolong the patient's disease process.

A patient with any type of disease should abstain from sex. If sex were continued perhaps no doctor in this world would be able to bring about a cure. Sex would rob the patient of the energy needed to help him or her get well.

A patient in pain should avoid both sour-tasting food and cold food. The sour taste enters the liver, the liver controls the nerves, and the liver, with added sour taste, will become stronger, thereby tightening the nerves and increasing the pain. Cold foods and drinks should be avoided because at the painful sites the arteries and veins will constrict, causing lowered blood supply to the area and increased pain. Cold foods in general will decrease the body's circulation, thus increasing pain. During painful diseases, the patient should also avoid indulging in anger to avoid increasing the pain.

A patient with skin disease or itching on the skin should avoid spicy food. This taste goes into the lungs. Since the lungs control the skin, with more spice, there will be more itching, and more small boils or abscesses will form.

A patient with carbuncles or skin ulcers should avoid eating rooster meat, as it will make the carbuncle worse. They should also avoid goose, carp, shrimp, crab, and any fish without scales. These foods will worsen the carbuncle or ulcer condition. If there is any pus in the carbuncle or ulcer, avoid peanuts, yellow beans, fatty pork, eggs, and sesame, since these foods will increase the amount of pus.

A patient with a cold or flu, or nose problems, should avoid chicken, goose, duck fatty meats, pork, and rice. Chicken is the worst, as it will increase the coughing or stuffed nose problems, and will prolong the fever. A patient with the flu should avoid *baht choi*, a Chinese vegetable dried under the sun and cooked with meat, which is usually good for the lungs. If eaten while the patient suffers from the flu, the disease will go inside the lungs. Duck will cause the flu to penetrate deeper into the body, prolonging any feverish condition. Deep-fried foods will increase the fever. Rice, because of its high starch content and subsequent glucose breakdown, will add fuel to the fever.

Patients with hypertension should avoid overheating foods, broiled or roasted foods, should decrease meat consumption and avoid alcohol, coffee, tobacco, salt, and teas containing caffeine.

Patients with heart problems should avoid alcohol, spicy foods, deep-fried foods, and strenuous activities such as climbing stairs and hard labor.

Patients with lung problems such as tonsillitis, bronchitis, coughing, asthma, and tuberculosis, should avoid sour, spicy, cold, fatty, and deep fried foods, *low baht* (white carrot), tobacco and alcohol.

Overcooling asthmatics should avoid vegetables, fruits, and cold foods.

Patients with stomach and intestinal problems should avoid foods that are difficult to digest (steak, roast beef, etc.), eggs, cakes made with eggs, sweet rice, sweet potatoes, *low baht,* sour foods, and cold foods.

Patients with inflammation in the kidneys should avoid overheating foods; patients with extreme dropsical conditions originating from kidney problems should avoid salt, fruit, and vegetables.

Patients with malaria should avoid cold foods, vegetables, and fruit, for one-half to one month until the condition abates.

Patients with cholera should not eat ginger, rice, cold foods, vegetables, or fruits. Patients with overcooling diseases should not eat cold foods, vegetables, and fruits. Patients with overheating diseases should not eat deep-fried or spicy foods.

鍼灸醫學全科

IV

Treatment of Specific Conditions

Headache

Causes: Catching cold; reading too much; neuralgia of the head. Neuralgia headaches may be chronic, occurring daily for many years, and are usually untreatable by Western medicine.

Symptoms: Headaches may occur on top of the head, over the whole head, on the back of the head, along the forehead, on the side of the head (as is the case with migraines), or as a painful point somewhere on the head. In addition, they may occur at a specific time of the day. Each kind of headache calls for a specific treatment, and is listed below as a distinct disorder.

Generalized Headache		
Principal points	Assistant Points	Auxiliary Points
GB-20, ST-8	LI-4, LU-7, GV-24, GV-20	GV-16, BL-10, BL-60, TW-1, GB-21, KI-1 XF-2 *(Tai Yang)* GV-4

Treatment

• ***Mild Headaches***

Use needle with mild stimulus on GB-20 and ST-8.

• ***Severe Headaches***

To draw down the blood and to quiet the nerves in the head, first apply the needle to LI-4 and LU-7, then apply the needle to GB-20, GV-16, and ST-8. Obtain a strong stimulus from points very distal to the head, and a light stimulus from points on the head. Some of the assistant points are used frequently, particularly GV-16, BL-10, and XF-2 *(Tai Yang)*. If the headache starts at the same time every day, bleed the finger or toe point corresponding to the meridian that is active at that time.

• ***Treatment of Headaches in Overheated Patients, with symptoms including a red face and a strong pulse***

After applying the treatment for severe headache, use a triangular needle on PC-9 and TW-1. Draw a few drops of blood from each point on both hands. If the patient does not respond, apply needles to GV-4 and KI-1, or use a triangular needle on GV-20 to draw a few drops of blood.

• ***Treatment of Headaches in Overcooled Patients, with symptoms including a pale face and a weak or slow pulse***

Use the treatment for severe headaches, as well as indirect moxa with ginger on GV-24 and GV-20. If the patient does not respond, apply 5 direct moxa (red bean size) to these points, and continue with 3 to 5 daily treatments. Alternately, use direct moxa (red bean size) 5-10 times on GV-4.

• ***Treatment of Headache in the Back of the Head***

Headache in the Back of the Head		
Principal Points	Assistant Points	Auxiliary Points
GB-20, GV-16, GV-19	LI-4, LU-7, GV-20	BL-10, XN-1 *(Pak Loh)*

Treatment

Step One: Apply needle to LI-4 and LU-7.

Step Two: Apply needle to GB-20, GV-16 and GV-19.

Step Three: Apply indirect moxa (with either an instrument or on ginger) to GV-19 and GV-20.

If the patient has a little headache after the preceding treatment, apply needle to *Pak Loh* and BL-10.

Note: For special conditions of headache in the back of head, see **Prognosis** and **Special Note** in the following section.

• *Treatment of Headache in the Forehead*

Headache in the Forehead		
Principal points	Assistant Points	Auxiliary Points
GV-16, ST-8, GV-23, GV-15 GV-24, LI-4	LI-11, BL-2, TW-23, GB-13 XF-2 *(Tai Yang)* XH-2	*Faht Jei*†, TW-21, GB-14

† At the front hairline on the Governing Vessel line.

Treatment

Step One: Apply needle to LI-4 and LI-11.

Step Two: Apply needle to GB-20, ST-8 and GV-23.

Step Three: If a headache is not of the overheating type, apply indirect moxa by ginger on GV-24. If the headache is very severe, apply direct moxa (1/2 rice size) to *Faht Jei,* (XH-4).

Step Four: If there is a little headache in the corner of the hairline after steps 1 to 3, needle GB-13. If there is a little headache in the temple region after steps 1 to 3, needle XF-2. If there is a little headache just over the eyebrows, use GB-14.

• *Treatment of Headache in One Side of the Head — Migraine*

Headache in One Side of the Head		
Principal points	Assistant Points	Auxiliary Points
ST-8, GB-20, GV-16, BL-2, XF-2 *(Tai Yang)*	LI-4, LU-7, GV-23, TW-23	KI-1, GV-4

Treatment

Step One: Apply needle to LI-4 and LU-7.

Step Two: Apply needle to GB-20, GV-16, ST-8, GV-23, BL-2, and TW-23.

Step Three: Apply needle to XF-2 and let the needle stay in the point for about 10 minutes.

Step Four: If the patient is empty or overcooling, continue with 3 direct moxa to XF-2 after needling. If the patient is full or overheating, do not apply moxa. Use the auxiliary points.

Note 1: The needle is to be applied bilaterally to both hand and leg points. However, treat the head points on the affected side only.

Note 2: When needling on the front of the scalp, slant the needle so that it moves parallel with the nose. On the upper back scalp, slant the needle to enter the head in the opposite direction. For GV-20, angle the needle in the direction of the pain. You may also control the direction of the stimulus by the angle of the needle.

Special Note: Overheated patients with headache, fever, no sensation of cold, and chronic constipation should be asked to take a purgative to facilitate recovery.

Prognosis: If the headache is mild, 1 to 3 treatments will be sufficient. More than 10 treatments may be required for chronic problems.

Anemia of the Brain

Causes: This illness may be either acute or chronic. *Acute anemia of the brain* is caused by a sudden loss of blood from the head. This may be created by sudden fright, severe pain, great anger, overwork, or hunger. These conditions cause a sudden weakening of the heart, and the patient may faint suddenly, losing consciousness.

Chronic anemia of the brain is caused by a gradual weakening of the heart and the body. The patient will tire easily and will always be drowsy, with headache, dizziness, and ringing in the ears. Loss of memory often accompanies this condition.

Treatment

• *Treatment of Acute Anemia of the Brain (Shock)*

Acute Anemia of the Brain	
Principal points	Assistant Points
GV-26, LU-11, LI-1 PC-9, TW-1, HT-9, SI-1	ST-36, KI-1, GV-24 GV-20

Step One: Apply needles to GV-26, LU-11, PC-9, LI-1, TW-1, HT-9 and SI-1, one after the other. Note that these are all very painful points, used to help the patient regain consciousness. If after treating one or two points the patient regains consciousness, there is no need to continue treatment.

Step Two: If after applying needles to all the points listed in the first step the patient does not regain consciousness, apply 3-5 direct moxa, or indirect moxa with ginger, to GV-24 and GV-20, and needle ST-36 and KI-1.

• *Treatment of Chronic Anemia of the Brain*

Chronic Anemia of the Brain		
Principal points	Assistant Points	Auxiliary Points
GB-20, GV-16, GV-24 GV-20	LI-4, LU-7, HT-7, ST-36, BL-18, GV-23 BL-10, BL-2	GV-22, GV-21, ST-8, GV-11 BL-15, GV-4 BL-38

Step One: Apply needle to LI-4, LU-7, and HT-7.

Step Two: Apply needle to GB-20, GV-16, and BL-10.

Step Three: Apply needle to GV-23 and BL-2.

Step Four: Apply indirect moxa with ginger once to GV-24 and GV-20 (only one application with each treatment).

If the illness proves difficult to cure, consider using steps one through three each day in combination with 5 direct moxa on GV-24 and GV-20. If the patient is very weak, apply five moxa to BL-15, GV-11, and BL-38. Use all three points for each of five consecutive treatments.

Prognosis: With acute anemia of the brain, one treatment should suffice. With chronic cases, 5 to 10 treatments should be sufficient. If the body is very weak, 20 to 30 treatments may be necessary.

Congestion of the Brain

Causes: Overexcitement; sunstroke.

Symptoms: Red, flushed face; the pulses of the neck and temple region are full and sometimes visible; headache; dizziness; ringing in the ears; dimness of vision. Persons 40 to 60 years of age are most susceptible to this illness, although patients who are 70 or older may also suffer from these symptoms.

Congestion of the Brain		
Principal Points	Assistant Points	Auxiliary Points
PC-9, SP-1, KI-1, BL-54 GV-14, GV-4, GV-20	LI-4, LU-7, LU-11, LI-1, LI-11, GB-20 SP-6, ST-36	PC-8, GV-22 GB-15, GV-23

Treatment

Step One: Apply needle to LI-4, LU-7 and LI-11.

Step Two: Apply needle to ST-36, SP-6, SP-1, KI-1 and BL-54.

Step Three: Apply needle to GB-20 and GV-14.

Step Four: Apply triangular needle to GV-20 and PC-9 and from each point withdraw a few drops of blood.

Step Five: When the blood pressure drops, apply 5-7 moxa to SP-6 during each treatment for 6 days and then regularly once a week. Continue for two months and the blood pressure will not rise again.

Prognosis: Mild conditions require 5 to 7 treatments. Serious conditions require 10 to 20 treatments.

Stroke
Cardiovascular Accident
Apoplexy

Causes: Congestion of the brain; arteriosclerosis of the brain.

Symptoms: Sudden fainting, or gradual loss of consciousness.

Special diagnosis: The presence of the following symptoms during a stroke indicates that the patient will die. *Do not treat a stroke victim if*:

- The pupils of the eyes enlarge
- The face is pale and white
- The mouth cannot be opened
- The jaw is locked open and cannot close
- There are signs of incontinence
- The eyeballs do not move
- There is phlegm or foam in the throat that gurgles and sounds like the drawing of a saw
- The pulse at the wrists feels like a straight pencil, moving uniformly up and down (beating at the three positions uniformly), or the pulse is very strong

Treatment

Treatment is best given as soon as possible, and if necessary can be given twice a day. Four conditions of apoplexy may be identified, with special treatments for each.

• ***Condition I, Treatment of Apoplexy, in which the patient's face is red and the pulse is strong:***

Step One: Apply needle to GV-26.

Step Two: Use triangular needle and draw a few drops of blood from GV-20.

Step Three: Apply triangular needle to LU-11, LI-1, PC-9, TW-1, HT-9 and SI-1. Use strong stimulus and draw out a few drops of blood from each point.

Step Four: Apply needle to LI-4, LI-11, LI-15, and KI-1. The patient will then recover. If during the course of applying the needle the patient awakens, discontinue further applications of the needle.

• ***Condition II, Treatment of Apoplexy, in which the patient has had a stroke and is still unconscious, but the face is not red and the pulse is soft and slow:***

Step One: Apply 3 direct moxa (red bean size) on GV-20.

Step Two: Apply needle to GV-26, LI-4, LI-11, LI-15, KI-1.

Note: If the patient wakes up through acupuncture treatment, this indicates that the hemiplegia was not severe. If, however, the patient wakes up by him or herself, this indicates that the hemiplegia was severe. Generally, the longer the patient takes to regain consciousness, the more severe the hemiplegia.

• ***Condition III, Treatment of Apoplexy, in which there is paralysis of one side of the face after the patient regains consciousness:***

Step One: Apply needle to LI-4, LU-7, and GV-26.

Step Two: Apply needle to GB-2, ST-6, ST-4, and CV-24. Electric stimulation may be used on all these points for five minutes.

Step Three: Apply indirect moxa with ginger or by use of an instrument to the points of the second step until the skin is reddish. If the patient does not respond well, use the "God's Needle" (Nim Ying moxa pole) to the points of the second step. Do not use direct moxa on the face unless the patient has been paralyzed for more than one year.

Auxiliary points: ST-8, GV-15, BL-2, TW-17, LI-20

Note: If paralysis of the face is present, but not associated with apoplexy, apply 3 direct moxa (green bean size) on GV-20 before the needle treatment.

If the muscles of the face turn to one side, treat the other side. Sometimes when the face is paralyzed, the muscles of the affected side are drawn down out of place, and it is difficult to decide which side of the face is affected. In order to determine this, tell the patient to laugh; she or he will only be able to move the normal side. The paralyzed side must then be treated. For paralysis of one side of the face use face points only on the paralyzed side, but use the points on the arms and hands bilaterally.

Another way to diagnose paralysis of the face is to tell the patient to blow from the mouth. The side from which the air comes out is the paralyzed side.

• ***Condition IV, Treatment of Apoplexy, in which the patient wakes up by him or herself after the stroke, or has been awake for a long time, and then comes for acupuncture treatment for the hemiplegia, and where the pulse is neither strong nor fast:***

Step One: Burn 3 direct moxa (red bean size) on GV-20 before proceeding with any other treatment. This will strengthen the nerves of the brain that control the body. If this is not done, subsequent treatment will not be as effective. If the patient's pulse is strong and fast after having awakened from a stroke, this indicates that his or her body is still "overheated." In this case, first get the stimulus at GV-20 with the triangular needle and then express a few drops of blood. If necessary, press the blood out with the fingers.

Step Two: **Treatment to arm and hand**: Apply needle to LI-15, LI-11, LI-10, TW-5, and LI-4, and then apply indirect moxa with ginger or instrument to these points.

Step Three: **Treatment to leg and foot**: Apply needle to BL-54, GB-30, GB-31, GB-34, ST-36, GB-39, and BL-60. Follow with indirect moxa with ginger or moxa instrument to these points, as to the arm. However, bear in mind that direct moxa must in no circumstances be applied to BL-54.

If the patient has awakened only within the month, and the pulse is still strong and fast, do not apply moxa after needles have been applied. Rather, apply electrical stimulation for five minutes, and then follow with indirect moxa.

If it has been longer than one month since the patient awoke from a stroke, if there is no ''overheating'' in the body and if the pulse is soft after needles have been applied, continue with indirect moxa or the ''God's Needle.''

If the paralysis does not respond to one week of daily treatment, and there is no overheating of the body, use direct moxa on all these points, using a few at a time, commencing with LI-15 and LI-11. This applies to any form of paralysis, whether preceded by apoplexy or not.

If paralysis has existed for a long time (over two years), and the patient's muscles are shortened so that the arm is flexed, needle PC-3, PC-7, and LU-5. If the leg muscles are shortened and flexed, use needle on BL-31, BL-32, BL-33, BL-34, and BL-23. However, when the muscles are flexed in this manner it must be borne in mind that it will be very difficult to cure the patient.

Prognosis: If none of the conditions noted under **Special Diagnosis (Apoplexy)** are present, then the apoplexy can be cured. In mild conditions, the patient will wake up after one or two treatments. In mild conditions of paralysis of the face, the patient will recover after 4 to 7 daily treatments. In the case of mild hemiplegia, 20 to 30 treatments will bring about recovery. Severe cases require longer treatments.

Prescription for Hemiplegia		
Herb		Quantity
Chinese	Pharmaceutical Name	
1. 北芪	*Radix Huangchi*	40g
2. 紅花	*Flos Carthami*	9g
3. 歸尾	*Angelica Sinensis*	9g
4. 川芎	*Rhizoma Ligustici*	9g
5. 地龍	*Lumbricus*	9g
6. 桃仁	*Semen Persicae*	9g
7. 赤芍	*Radix Paeonia Lactiflora*	9g

Boil the above prescription in five cups of water until one cup remains. Drink when warm. If the patient is overheating, reduce herb #1 to 10 grams; if the patient's body is overcooling, reduce herbs #2 and #3 to 3 grams. Two doses over the course of one week will help give mobility to the arm and leg. If the patient has taken the prescription three times and there is no effect, discontinue use.

The traditional Chinese pharmacist uses the *Ch'ien* (錢) (equal to approximately 3 grams) as the basic unit for weighing herbs in prescriptions.

Water in the Head — Hydrocephalus

Causes: Hydrocephalus may occur as a *prenatal* or *postnatal* condition. *Prenatal hydrocephalus* occurs when water enters the infant's skull while in utero. *Postnatal hydrocephalus* may occur as a result of meningitis, an injury to the head, a carbuncle or abscess, or surgery on the scalp.

Symptoms: When this condition is seen in an infant, the face of the baby will be very small, while the head is the size of an adult's. The baby appears to be very stupid, and the eyes always look downwards. In prenatal conditions, children generally do not live more than one or two years, dying of cramp. In postnatal hydrocephalus, the child may live 4-5 years, although death usually occurs earlier.

Postnatal hydrocephalus also occurs in adults, and is much easier to cure than the prenatal variety. One patient of mine was a man of 40 who had a growth removed from his skull by surgery. Immediately following the operation, the skull began to swell from the middle top of the skull to the skin of the temples. The patient's condition was cured after burning moxa on GV-24 and GV-20, and applying needles to LI-4, LU-7, GB-20, GV-16, GV-20, and XF-3 *(Yin Tang)*.

Treatment

Step One: Apply needle to XF-2 *(Tai Yang)*, BL-54, PC-3, LU-11, LI-1, PC-9, HT-9, and SI-1. In all the above-mentioned points draw out blood after acupuncture.

Step Two: Apply needle to LI-4, LI-11, LU-5, ST-8, GB-20, GV-16, and GV-26.

Step Three: Apply direct moxa on GV-24 and GV-20. Continue daily for about 5 days, 5 moxa on each point. For a baby, use 1/2 rice grain size moxa. For an adult, use red bean size moxa.

Prognosis: Postnatal cases of hydrocephalus are easy to cure. However, prenatal cases are difficult to help unless treatment is given early enough.

Madness or Mania

Causes: Heredity; overwork; drunkenness; frustration; high fever over a long period of time.

Symptoms: Talking or doing nonsense; crying or singing at inappropriate times; great anger or fear; disorientation and the inability to recognize familiar people. Some patients may not feel hungry and do not eat for long periods of time. Raving patients always climb up to a high place to sing or run along the road, or pick up a knife to kill somebody.

Madness or Mania		
Principal points	Assistant Points	Auxiliary Points
GV-26, GV-16, GV-20, PC-7, GV-24 HT-7, PC-5, SI-3, SP-1	PC-8, LI-11, GV-23, BL-15, GV-1	GB-20, GV-15, ST-42, XH-2 *(Sen Chung)*, CV-14, LI-5

Treatment

When madness is caused by high fever and constipation, apply needles to LU-11, PC-9, and to all 10 fingertip points. Press each to draw blood. Then, needle LI-4, LI-11, GV-14, BL-12, GB-20, LV-14, KI-1 and BL-54.

For idiocy and stupidity: Apply needle to HT-7, PC-7, PC-5, LU-11, CV-12, KI-1, BL-54, and GV-20. Apply 5 moxa to GV-20.

Prognosis: For mild cases, a few treatments will suffice; for severe cases, about 20 treatments will be required.

The Thirteen Ghost Points for Madness by Sun Szi Miao, 618 A.D.

The 13 Ghost points	
1. Ghost Palace	GV-26
2. Ghost Letter	LU-11
3. Ghost Castle	SP-1
4. Ghost Heart	PC-7
5. Ghost Road	BL-62†
6. Ghost Pillow	GV-16
7. Ghost Bed	ST-6
8. Ghost Market	CV-24
9. Ghost Cave	PC-8
10. Ghost Hall	GV-23
11. Ghost Hidden	CV-1
12. Ghost Leg	LI-11†
13. Ghost Seal	XF-7

† Use fire needle

Treating cases of madness by needling the above points in the order listed will be most effective.

Epilepsy (Seizures)

Causes: This disease is usually inherited. It can also come from excessive drinking or excessive sexual intercourse. Sometimes it is caused by worry or anxiety. Usually it will start before the patient is twenty.

Symptoms: This disease will appear suddenly as unconsciousness, with total body cramps. The face becomes pale, the lips blue. Sometimes the artery above the umbilical cord will jump. Usually the patient will make noises like a lamb and will exude saliva. Seizure occurs in four steps:

1. The patient falls and becomes unconscious
2. The body becomes very rigid
3. The body undergoes convulsions
4. The patient wakes up

Even without treatment, the patient will wake up within 1-3 minutes. While unconscious, the patient will clench his or her teeth, bite his or her tongue, hit his or her own body, lose semen and feces. When the patient awakens there is no memory of what happened.

In another condition the epileptic fit is similar to a stroke. There is still body cramping, unconsciousness lasts longer and there is congestion in the brain. When the patient wakes up, there is hemiplegia.

Treatment

The following treatments may be used alone or in combination to treat epilepsy.

Do not treat the patient during a seizure; treat the patient *between* seizures only.

- ***Treatment I for Epilepsy:***

Apply needle to PC-5, PC-7, PC-8, SI-3, GV-26, CV-12, KI-6 (if the seizure occurs at night use 5 moxa on this point), and BL-62 (if the seizure happens in the daytime use 5 moxa on this point).

• *Treatment II for Epilepsy:*

Apply 5 green bean size moxa, or indirect moxa, every day on GV-24, GV-20, GV-14, BL-22, CV-15, CV-14 and KI-1.

• *Treatment III for Epilepsy:*

Apply direct moxa on BL-13, BL-20, and PC-5. Use moxa green bean size. Apply needle to SI-3, HT-7, BL-60, BL-63 and KI-6. Do this every 3 days for two months.

• *Treatment IV for Epilepsy:*

During the time of the seizure, apply moxa to KI-1, CV-12, and the Ghost Crying point. Bind the patient's thumbs together, and burn a big piece of moxa between the two thumbs in the area between the nail and the skin. After the patient wakes up, the seizures that follow will be less severe.

Auxiliary points: GV-22, SP-1, and BL-38.

Note: According to the old book, direct moxa should not be applied on the first treatment. A purgative should be given to cause diarrhea a day prior to using direct moxa. If this isn't done, the condition will be worse than before.

Prognosis: If the problem starts either before the age of 10 or during middle age, it is difficult to cure. If the problem starts when the patient is 15-20 years old, the prognosis is better. Males are easier to treat than females. Twenty to thirty treatments should be given.

Neurasthenia

Causes: Overwork; oversmoking, irregular meals; internal organ poisoning; masturbation.

Symptoms: Neurasthenia usually occurs during middle age. The illness is divided into *cranial nerve type (vagus nerve)*, *spinal nerve type (sympathetic)* and *mixed type.*

Cranial-type neurasthenia is usually caused by emotional disturbance. The face is flushed, patient complains of heaviness of head and headache, loses concentration and understanding in reading, often suffers from insomnia, is easily delighted and provoked, has sudden changes in temperament, is often frightened and has palpitations, rapid pulse, loss of appetite, and habitual constipation.

Spinal-type neurasthenia is also caused by emotional disturbance, but the face is anemic and pale, the pulse slow, the patient has bronchial and esophageal spasm, vomiting and diarrhea, frequent urination, general aching, feels fatigue in the muscles upon awakening, more muscular fatigue of lower limbs when walking, and complains of aching in the sacral region and tenderness of the spine.

Treatment

• *Treatment of Cranial-Type Neurasthenia*

Cranial Type Neurasthenia		
Principal Points	Assistant Points	Auxiliary Points
GB-20, HT-7, GV-24, GV-20	LI-4, LU-7, ST-36	CV-15, GV-11, GB-21, BL-38

Step One Apply needle to LI-4, LU-7 and HT-7.

Step Two Apply needle to GB-20 and ST-36.

Step Three Apply moxa to GV-24 and GV-20.

• *Treatment of Sympathetic-Type Neurasthenia*

Sympathetic-Type Neurasthenia		
Principal Points	Assistant Points	Auxiliary Points
BL-18, BL-20, BL-24, GV-4	BL-31, BL-32, BL-33, BL-34 CV-12, ST-36	CV-15, GV-11 GV-21, BL-38

Step One: Apply needle and then moxa on all principle points.

Step Two: Apply needle and moxa on all assistant points.

Note: For mixed-type neurasthenia, use points and methods from the above treatments according to the presenting symptoms.

Prognosis: For mild cases about 10 treatments; severe cases about 30 treatments.

Sleep Disorders

Insomnia

Internal Causes: Fever; pain; itching; digestive disturbance; overeating or drinking before going to bed; disturbance in the circulatory/ respiratory systems; overwork.

Emotional causes: Nervous disorders; nervous weakness; sexual disturbance; too much thinking before going to bed.

External causes: Noise; changes of weather.

Symptoms: Restlessness; worrying; anxiety; shallow sleep; short sleep; weariness. A long period of such illness will cause central nervous fatigue and may even cause death.

Treatment of Insomnia

Insomnia		
Principal Points	Assistant Points	Auxiliary Points
HT-7, BL-13 LU-9, SP-1	SP-6, SP-9, KI-6, HT-6, PC-6	HT-4, PC-5, BL-54, BL-8

Note 1: It is advisable to perform treatment just before patient goes to bed.

Note 2: If insomnia is caused by overcooling of the brain, use 5 moxa on GV-20.

Prognosis For new cases, about 2 treatments will suffice, and for long-standing cases about 10 treatments will be needed.

Oversleeping

Apply needle on HT-7, LI-13, KI-6, KI-4, KI-3, SP-5, KI-1, and BL-12. Apply moxa on GV-22, GV-24 and GV-11.

Trigeminal Neuralgia — Pain of the Face —

Causes: Catching cold; injury to the face; trigeminal neuralgia caused by diseases of the eyes, ears, nose, or teeth.

Symptom: Severe neuralgia of the face.

The trigeminal nerve has three distinct branches. The first branch enervates the forehead and eyebrows. The second branch travels to the ear, under the eyes, along the nose and finally to the upper lip. The third branch runs down from the ear to the jaw and eventually to the corner of the lip. Treatment of trigeminal neuralgia will be determined by the branch affected.

Treatment

• *Treatment of First Branch Trigeminal Neuralgia*

Trigeminal Neuralgia; First Branch		
Principal points	Assistant Points	Auxiliary Points
ST-8, BL-2, TW-23	LI-4, LI-11 GB-20 TW-21,	GV-24, GV-23, XF-1 *(San Cha)* GB-15

Step One: Apply needle to LI-4 and LI-11.

Step Two: Apply needle to ST-8, BL-2, and TW-23.

• ***Treatment of Second Branch Trigeminal Neuralgia***

Trigeminal Neuralgia; Second Branch		
Principal points	Assistant Points	Auxiliary Points
GB-2, LI-20, ST-6	LI-4, LI-11	XF-1 *(San Cha)*

Step One: Apply needle to LI-4 and LI-11.

Step Two: Apply needle to GB-2, ST-6, and LI-20

• ***Treatment of Third Branch Trigeminal Neuralgia***

Trigeminal Neuralgia; Third Branch		
Principal points	Assistant Points	Auxiliary Points
ST-6, ST-4, CV-24	LI-4, LI-11 XF-1 *(San Cha)*	

Step One: Apply needle to LI-4 and LI-11.

Step Two: Apply needle to ST-6, ST-4, and CV-24.

Note 1: If two or three branches are simultaneously affected, then all the points mentioned may be needled. Follow this with indirect moxa by instrument or ginger to all points except those where the use of moxa is prohibited: BL-2, TW-23, ST-8, and LI-20.

Note 2: Five direct moxa on XF-1 *(San Cha)* is very effective.

Prognosis: For mild conditions, 3 to 5 treatments will be required. For severe conditions, up to about 10 treatments may be necessary.

Acute Inflammation of the Conjunctiva with Catarrh — Conjunctivitis —

Causes: Dust; chemical vapors; strong light; bacteria or germs.

Symptoms: The conjunctiva and eyeballs are inflamed and swollen, and there is itchiness and a feeling of something being in the eye, with little pain.

Conjunctivitis		
Principal points	Assistant Points	Auxiliary Points
XF-2, ST-8, BL-2, BL-1	LI-4, LI-11, TW-23, GB-15, GB-1	GB-20, BL-18, GV-4, XF-4 *(Yu Yao)*† TW-1, GV-23

† At the middle of the eyebrows

Treatment

Step One: Apply needle to LI-4 and LI-11.

Step Two: Apply needle to ST-8, GB-15, BL-2, TW-23, and GB-1.

Step Three: Apply needle to BL-1. Because this is a painful point, use it as the last point of needle application. In general, it is wise to apply needle to the painful points last.

Step Four: If, after the first 3 steps, the inflammation still remains, it may be because the inflammation is in the region of the temple. In this case, needle XF-2. Alternatively, apply the needle to XF-4 *(Yu Yao)*. Squeeze out a few drops of blood from *Yu Yao*. The inflammation will cease in a few hours to one day. One may also bleed the vein on the back of the ear to achieve the same result.

Step Five: If there is headache caused by this illness, apply the needle to GB-20.

Step Six: If there is trachoma in the conjunctiva, in addition to the first three steps, apply needle to BL-20 and BL-21. The patient will then recover.

Step Seven: Find a red spot on the back and bleed it. This will also give good results.

Step Eight: In conditions that include the inability to close the eye, apply needle to BL-1, ST-4, and GB-1.

Step Nine: In conditions including eye pain, apply needle to LI-4, LI-11, ST-8, BL-2, and BL-1.

Note: Since traditional Chinese medical theory teaches that the upper eyelid is affected by the spleen and the lower eyelid by the stomach, Chinese doctors believe that trachoma is due to *Supp* of the spleen and stomach. To produce such a condition, the *Supp* must have been present for a long period of time, perhaps as long as several years.

Prognosis: For acute inflammation of the conjunctiva, two to three treatments are necessary. For trachoma, 10 to 20 treatments are required.

Chronic Inflammation of the Tear Duct

Causes: The tube of the tear duct may be too narrow, thus inhibiting drainage; some germs or bacteria may be in the tear duct; or the liver is "empty" or weak, resulting in insufficient blood in the liver.

Treatment

• *Condition I, in which the eyes water when wind blows on them:*

Step One: Apply needle to LI-4, GB-20, ST-8, and GB-15.

Step Two: Apply needle to BL-1.

Step Three: Apply 7 direct moxa (1/2 rice grain size) to *Dah guu Kung,* and the next day apply 7 direct moxa on *Shiao guu Kung.* If after the first day's treatment the eyes cease to water, there will be no need to apply direct moxa to *Shiao guu Kung* on the second day.

Prognosis: About 3 to 5 treatments will be necessary for recovery.

• *Condition II, in which one or both eyes are constantly watery:*

Step One: Apply needle to SI-3, GB-20, and BL-2.

Step Two: Apply 7 direct moxa (red bean size) on BL-18.

Continue the above treatment for 3 days. On the 4th day and on the next 3 days, apply 5 direct moxa (green bean size) on GV-20, while continuing with the same needle application. If the condition has not improved after 6 days, apply direct moxa 7 times (1/2 rice grain size) alternating between *Dah guu Kung* and *Shiao guu Kung.*

Prognosis: About 3 to 10 treatments will be necessary for complete recovery.

Inability to Open the Eyelids

Causes: Severe migraine headache or eye disease.

Symptoms: The eyelids are closed and cannot open of themselves.

Treatment

Step One: Apply needle to LI-4 and LI-11 bilaterally.

Step Two: Apply needle to ST-8, GB-15, GB-20, GB-1, and BL-1 of the affected side.

Step Three: Apply needle to *Yu Yao* on the affected side. First put in the needle and c tain the stimulus. Withdraw the needle and when nearly at the surface direct the needle to BL-2 and obtain the stimulus from that point. Withdraw the needle again almost to the surface and direct the needle to TW-23 and obtain the stimulus from the point. Withdraw the needle completely.

Prognosis: In mild cases, one treatment will be sufficient. In severe conditions, 3 or more treatments may be required.

Night Blindness

Causes: Lack of nourishment (vitamin A); weakness of the nerves of the body; sequelae of jaundice or childbirth, when the mother is very weak. Chinese doctors believe this condition is due to emptiness of the liver.

Symptoms: Inability to see without direct sunlight. Even in artificial light, the patient is unable to see.

Treatment

Step One: Apply needle to GV-23, GV-20, BL-23, and GV-4.

Step Two: Apply needle to BL-18. Directly after applying needle to BL-18, apply direct moxa 7 times (red bean size) to that point. If the patient feels that the pain is too great, apply indirect moxa with ginger to BL-18.

Step Three: Apply 5 direct moxa (green bean size) to GV-24, or indirect moxa with ginger to GV-24.

Step Four: Apply needle to BL-1.

Note: If the patient is very weak, recovery may not be possible with the above treatment alone. In these cases, apply 5 direct moxa (red bean size) to BL-38, and 3 direct moxa to ST-36 and GB-20. Auxiliary points include BL-2 and GB-20.

Prognosis: 3 to 5 treatments will suffice.

Prescription for Night Blindness	
Step One	Mix 9 grams each of Semen Cassia Torae and Excrementum Vespertilii with 4 ounces of pig liver.
Step Two	Boil the above mixture in 3 cups of water until 1 cup remains.
Step Three	Have the patient drink when warm, once a day fo 3 days. The liver may also be eaten to good effect.

Cataract

Causes: Chinese doctors say that this is due to "overheating" of the liver, and "overcooling" and "emptiness" of the kidneys.

Symptoms: This is an ailment affecting elderly people, though sometimes persons about 30 years of age are affected. The patient is unable to see clearly, even in the daytime. Looking into his or her pupil you will see what looks like a tiny white cloud.

Treatment

Step One: Apply needle to LI-4, ST-36 and LV-2.

Step Two: Apply needle to GB-20 and BL-18.

Step Three: Apply needle to BL-2, GB-1, and BL-1.

Step Four: Apply 5 direct moxa (red bean size) to GV-4 and BL-23, one point the first day, one point the second.

Step Five: Apply indirect moxa with ginger on GV-24 and GV-20. If the patient is also suffering from ischemia of the brain, apply 5 direct moxa (red bean size) to GV-24 and GV-20.

Prognosis: In mild conditions, 2 weeks of daily treatment with Chinese medicines. In severe conditions, 1 to 2 months of daily treatments.

Prescription for Cataract		
Herb		Quantity
Chinese	Pharmaceutical Name	
熟地	*Radix Rehmanniae*	120g
菊花	*Flos Chrysanthemi*	90g
山藥	*Fructus Corni Officianalis*	60g
丹皮	*Cortex Mouton*	15g
炒澤瀉	*Rhizoma Alismatis*	15g
黃柏	*Cortex Phellodendri*	30g
知母	*Rhizoma Anemarrhenae*	30g
膽星	*Pulvis Arisaemae cum Felle Bovis*	60g
半夏	*Rhizoma Pinelliae*	60g
枸杞	*Fructus Lycii*	60g
楮實	*Fructus Broussonetiae*	60g
兔絲子	*Herba et Semen Cuscutae*	60g
蒺藜	*Fructus Tribuli*	60g
青箱子	*Semen Celosiae*	60g

Grind all of the above herbs into a powder and mix with high quality honey. The mixture should not be too wet or too dry. Make pills 3/4″ in diameter, then dry them in the oven. Do not over-dry. Take as a candy, three times a day, until recovered.

The traditional Chinese pharmacist uses the *Ch'ien* (錢) (equal to approximately 3 grams) as the basic unit for weighing herbs in prescriptions.

Minor Eye Problems

• ***The Eye Cannot Close:*** Apply needle on ST-4, GB-1, BL-1, and LI-4.

• ***Small Abscess on the Eyelid (Stye):*** Find a small red spot on the upper back, between the neck and BL-38. For an abscess on the left eye, treat the red spot on the right side of the back; for an abscess on the right eye, treat the red spot on the left side of the back. Use the triangular needle to pierce the red spot 1/8″ deep or a little deeper, and squeeze out some blood. After a few days the eyelid abscess will disappear and will not come back again.

• ***Pterygium:*** Pterygium is a muscle-like vasculature growing from canthus to iris. Apply needle to BL-18 and SI-1, and squeeze a few drops of blood. If the pterygium is on the inner canthus, add BL-1. If on the outer canthus, add GB-1. This case is easy to treat in the beginning. If the case is too old, it is difficult to get good results, although treatment will stop it from advancing.

Deafness

Causes: Weakness or overcooling of the body; injury by striking the head near the ear; an extremely loud sound close to the ear; inflammation of the middle ear.

Symptoms Sometimes the patient suddenly can hear and then suddenly becomes deaf again. Sometimes the patient is one who can hear loud sounds but not soft ones. In severe cases, patients are unable to hear at all.

Treatment

• ***Treatment of mild deafness, and in cases when the patient has become suddenly deaf:***

Step One: Apply needle to LI-1 (without drawing blood), SI-19, and GB-2.

Step Two: Use one-quarter to one-half inch pieces of *Chong Shu* (Atractylis Ovata), one side cut level and the other cut to a point. Wrap the pointed end in cotton wool and put this in the patient's ear. Burn 7-27 moxa (yellow bean size) on the flat tip of the *Chong Shu* and rest the head, lying down on the side of the head which is not being treated.

• ***Treatment of severe conditions of deafness, when the patient is unable to hear at all, or has been deaf for a very long time:***

Step One: Apply needle to TW-5, TW-3, and LI-1.

Step Two: Apply needle to TW-21, SI-19, GB-2, and TW-17. Insert all needles deeply (over one inch), and leave for half an hour. After the needles have been removed, use indirect moxa on all these points.

Step Three: Apply needle to BL-23 if the condition of the patient's kidney is "empty" or "overcooling." This can be determined by the pulse. After applying the needle, it is wise to apply 5-7 direct moxa (green bean size) to BL-23.

This treatment should be carried out daily for several days. Needling GB-20, SI-3, and LI-5 as assistant points is also recommended.

Prognosis: If the ear drum is not broken, the deafness can be easily cured. In acute deafness, or mild conditions, 3-7 treatments should suffice. In chronic deafness or severe conditions, daily treatment for three weeks to two months will be necessary.

Prescription for Deafness	
Step One	Place a tortoise on a clean pan and give it a look at itself by placing a mirror before it. This will induce the tortoise to urinate.
Step Two	Mix the tortoise urine with *Mui Pien* (Borneo camphor) powder. Use a small piece of cotton wool to absorb the mixture.
Step Three	Apply the soaked cotton to the hole of the ear when going to bed at night, and withdraw the next morning. After a few such applications to the ear, the patient's hearing will greatly improve.

Inflammation of the Middle Ear — Otitis Media —

Causes: Tears or water entering the ear; external injury to the ear; touching the inside of the ear.

Symptoms: Inflammation and pain in the ear, possibly with swelling of the face near the ear, occasionally with pus.

Treatment

• *Treatment of more severe conditions of Otitis Media*:

Step One: Apply needle to LI-4, LI-11, and ST-6.

Step Two: If the pain is very severe, apply indirect moxa with ginger to ST-6, GB-2, and SI-19.

Step Three: If the pain becomes mild after the first and second steps, apply needle to GB-2 and SI-19. Follow immediately with indirect moxa with ginger; the pain will then cease.

• *Treatment of other conditions involving Otitis Media*:

Step One: Apply needle to LI-4 and LI-11.

Step Two: Apply needle to ST-6, GB-2, and SI-19.

Step Three: Apply indirect moxa with ginger on ST-6, GB-2, and SI-19.

If there is a lot of pus inside the ear, use hydrogen peroxide or Chinese tea to wash away the pus, and then wash out the ear again with Rivenal water. Dry the ear with clean cotton wool, and then blow a little *Mui Pien* powder into the ear. If the inflammation of the ear is chronic, apply the needle to the 3 points of **Step Two**, and then apply 5 direct moxa (red bean size) on GB-2 on the affected side. Only one such treatment will be necessary. In one to two weeks the patient will recover completely.

Prognosis: In acute conditions, 1 to 3 treatments will be required; in chronic conditions, 1 treatment (as indicated above).

Ringing in the Ears

Causes: Diseases of the heart or kidneys; anemia.

Symptoms: Ringing in the ear like a bell, or hearing a constant sound of flowing water, knocking, roaring like a lion, insect singing, etc.

Treatment

Step One: Apply needle to GB-2, SI-19, TW-17, and GB-20.

Step Two: Apply needle to TW-2 and BL-23.

Step Three: Use *Chong Shu* (Atractylis Ovata) in the ear, as described above in the first treatment, **Step Two** for **Deafness**.

Step Four: If the condition is severe, apply 3 direct moxa (green bean size) to BL-15, BL-23, and GB-20. Apply direct moxa to one of these points for three to five days, then the second point for three to five days, and finally the third, until all three have been used.

• *Alternate Treatment*

Step One: Apply needles to GB-2, TW-17, TW-18, TW-19, and TW-22.

Step Two: Leave the needles in the points for half an hour. As the needles are removed, some effect should be noticed.

Assistant points: GV-4, LI-5, LI-1, and ST-36.

Prognosis: In mild conditions, 7 to 10 treatments are required. In severe or chronic conditions, more than 30 treatments will be necessary.

Note: Sometimes this case is very difficult to treat. Ear acupuncture is quite helpful, and should be considered in the treatment of tinnitis.

Ringing in the Ears with Severe Dizziness — Menier's Syndrome —

Causes: Neuritis of the nerve of the ear; chronic ear trouble; injury to the head.

Symptoms: Ringing in the ear with severe vertigo. The patient may experience ringing in the ears while very dizzy, and feel that everything is turning around. Sometimes the patient vomits and falls to the ground.

Treatment

Step One: Apply needle to XH-4 *(Faht Jei)* with rapid shallow pricking. Squeeze out a few drops of blood.

Step Two: Apply needle to ST-36, BL-62, and GB-20.

Step Three: Apply indirect moxa with ginger, or 3 direct moxa to GV-20, GV-24, and GV-23. If the patient has not recovered, apply 3 to 5 direct moxa (green bean size) to ST-36.

Assistant points: GV-4, BL-23, BL-22, and GB-21.

Prognosis: In acute conditions, 1-2 treatments will suffice. In chronic conditions, 5-10 treatments will be necessary. If the ear is still ringing, use the **Alternative Treatment** for **Ringing in the Ears**, above.

Mumps

Symptoms: This is most common among school children, and is highly infectious. Symptoms include swelling under the ear and in the region of the face and neck, with inflammation and minor pain.

Treatment

Step One: Apply needle to LI-4, LI-11 and ST-6.

Step Two: Apply needle to BL-54.

Step Three: If there is no fever, apply indirect moxa with ginger in the inflamed region. If there is fever, it is better not to apply moxa, but to apply a triangular needle to LU-11 and LI-1, and draw out a few drops of blood.

Prognosis: Three to five treatments will bring about recovery.

Lockjaw

Treatment

Step One: Apply needle to LI-4, and apply triangular needle to LU-11, drawing out a few drops of blood.

Step Two: Apply needle to GB-2, ST-6, and GV-26.

Acute Sinusitis

Causes: Catching cold, or getting wet in the rain in cold weather.

Symptoms: Sneezing; stuffed nose; loss of sense of smell; runny nose.

Treatment

Step One: Apply needle to LI-4.

Step Two: Apply needle to GB-20, GV-14, BL-12, LI-20, and XF-5 *(Pie Yin).*

If the condition is mild, the results obtained from the first and second steps alone will be satisfactory. In severe conditions, however, it would be advisable to needle GV-16, GV-26, and GV-25, and then continue with indirect moxa with ginger to BL-12 and GV-22.

Prognosis: In mild conditions, 1 treatment will suffice, and the result will be immediate. In chronic conditions, 3 treatments should suffice.

Chronic Sinusitis

Causes: Chronic colds, which, before recovery, are repeated by further attacks; smoking too much; overuse of alcoholic beverages, which may cause the blood vessels in the nose to become inflamed.

Symptoms: Chronic stuffed nose, which is most severe at night when in bed; chronic runny nose, often accompanied by an offensive smell from the patient's nose; loss of sense of smell; nasal speech.

Note: Before treating the patient, check the balance of the lungs and spleen with *akabane* (see Part I, chapter 5, section 5.2, ''Balancing the Sympathetic Nerves,'' above).

Treatment

Step One: Apply needle to LI-4, LI-20, and GV-25.

Step Two: Apply needle to GB-20, XN-1 *(Pak Loh),* GV-16, and BL-12.

Step Three: Apply 5 direct moxa (red bean size) to GV-22 or GV-24.

Continue the above treatment daily for 7 days. If the patient has not completely recovered after this time, substitute BL-12 and GV-23 or GV-22, applying 5 direct moxa (green bean size) to them, and continue the daily treatment until the patient recovers. Five direct moxa on BL-20 may also prove to be quite effective; however direct moxa is not to be applied to both points during one treatment.

Prognosis: 10-20 treatments should bring about a complete recovery.

Piles of the Nose — Polyps

Symptoms: A growth like a small bag appears, dropping from the inside of the nose, possibly filling up the nostril. The patient has a running nose and headache. The patient breathes through the mouth only. Either one nostril or both nostrils may be affected. Sometimes this condition appears simultaneously with asthma.

Treatment

Step One: Apply needle to LI-4 and LI-11.

Step Two: Apply needle to GB-20, GV-16, BL-12, GV-26, LI-20, XF-5 *(Pie Yen)* and GV-25.

Step Three: Apply 5 direct moxa times (green bean size) to GV-22 and GV-23.

Step Four: Use indirect moxa with ginger over the entire nose.

The above treatment should be continued until the polyps in the nose have been completely reduced.

Prognosis: If the polyps have just appeared, about 7 treatments will suffice. If they have been present for a few months or years, as many as 30 treatments may be necessary. In some cases, however, polyps of the nose cannot be cured by acupuncture and require surgery. After the surgery, acupuncture treatment would prevent the polyps from recurring.

Nose Bleeding — Epistaxis

Causes: Pneumonia; inflammation of the nose; high blood pressure; overheating of the body.

Treatment

• *Treatment of Chronic Nosebleeds*

Step One: Apply needle to LI-4 and LI-11.

Step Two: Apply needle to GV-14, GV-16, BL-12, BL-13, and LI-20.

Step Three: Apply 5 direct moxa (green bean size) to GV-23.

Assistant points: BL-60, GV-20, GV-15, KI-1, SI-3, and BL-54.

• *Treatment of Acute Nosebleeds*

Apply one ½ rice-grain size moxa to LI-11 on the oppposite side than the bleeding nostril; if blood is coming from both nostrils, apply bilaterally. The bleeding will cease immediately.

Prognosis: In acute conditions, 1 treatment will suffice. In chronic conditions, about 7 treatments are required.

Prescription for Epistaxis	
Step One	Take the skin off one large dry garlic.
Step Two	Pound the garlic and apply to KI-1, binding the garlic tightly to the skin. If the bleeding is from the left nostril, apply the garlic to KI-1 of the right foot; if bleeding is from the right nostril, apply the garlic to KI-1 of the left foot.

Toothache

Causes: Decay of the enamel of the tooth and exposure of the nerve; neuralgia of the nerve of the bone after tooth extraction; any disease in the area of the tooth; excessive eating of roasted, toasted, or other "overheating" foods, such as "hot" peppers or chilis; acute constipation; lack of sleep.

Symptoms: Toothache, with or without swelling of the jaw, causing inability to eat and sleep.

Treatment

• ***For Toothache in the Upper Jaw:*** Apply needle to LI-4, ST-44, ST-6, TW-21, and GV-26.

• ***For Toothache in the Lower Jaw:*** Apply needle to LI-4, ST-44, ST-6, and CV-24.

If the tooth is broken, after applying the needle apply indirect moxa with ginger on CV-24. Apply powdered *Wu Bei Zi* (Galla Sinensis) in the hole of the tooth.

If there is swelling of the jaw, apply indirect moxa with ginger on the place that is swollen. If you have found that the case is one of "overheating," however, do not use moxa.

If there is a small abscess close to or under the tooth, apply indirect moxa with ginger on CV-24. Applying 7 direct moxa to CV-24 is most effective in the case of an abscess in a tooth; the needle cannot adequately take the place of direct moxa for such cases. However, due to the likelihood of a scar from the moxa, do not apply direct moxa to this point unless absolutely necessary.

Osteomyelitis of the Jawbone

Causes: Chronic inflammation of the jawbone caused by tooth decay and germs getting into the bone.

Symptoms: Swelling of the jaw with some pain, with the mouth unable to open freely. Later, there is decay of the jawbone. The disease may advance very slowly, and may progress for as much as a few years before the patient dies from it.

Treatment

Step One:	Apply 6 direct moxa (green bean size) to CV-24.
Step Two:	If the condition is severe, follow **Step One** with 7 direct moxa (red bean size) to LI-4.
Step Three:	Apply indirect moxa with ginger or garlic to the region that is swollen.
Step Four:	Apply needle to LI-4, ST-6, ST-44, or 7 direct moxa on ST-6.

Prognosis: In early stages, this condition can be successfully cured by acupuncture and moxibustion treatment with 7 to 10 treatments. In late stages of lockjaw, when the jaw is very swollen and the teeth decayed, acupuncture will not be effective.

Bleeding of the Gums

Causes: Inflammation of the gums or jaw; diabetes; kidney disease; amenorrhea; overheating of the stomach.

Symptoms: The gums under the teeth bleed constantly. In acute cases, the gums bleed severely; in chronic cases, the bleeding is mild, and may be accompanied by a little pus.

Treatment

Step One: Apply needle to LI-4 and LI-10.

Step Two: Apply needle to ST-44 and KI-3.

Step Three: Apply needle to GV-16, CV-24, and ST-6.

Step Four: If the condition is acute and the body is "overheated," apply needle to XF-8 (*Jin Jin* and *Yu Yeh,* on the two veins under the surface of the tongue), and to LI-1, and express a few drops of blood from these points.

Step Five: If the condition is chronic, apply 7 direct moxa (green bean size) to ST-6 and CV-24, daily for a few days.

Prognosis: In acute or mild conditions, 1 or 2 treatments will be necessary. In chronic conditions, over 10 treatments will be required.

Prescription for Bleeding Gums
For acute cases, put the dregs of fresh bean curd in the mouth and keep it there until it becomes warm. Change several times for a fresh mouthful until the bleeding stops.

Exophthalmic Goiter

Causes: This illness is most common among 30 to 40 year old women, and may be accompanied by irregular menstruation, worrying about the future, or overwork.

Symptoms: The patient appears anemic, and suffers from palpitation of the heart, prominent eyeballs, and shaky arms and legs. The pulse is fast and the patient is short of breath. The gland of the neck is swollen. If this condition has continued for a long period, the heart will suffer, and the patient will die from generalized weakness.

Treatment

• ***On the first, fourth, and seventh days:***

Step One: Locate the points between the 4th and 5th and between the 5th and 6th cervical vertebrae on the center line of the spine. Then go one ''eye division'' lateral in both directions from each of these points. Four points will thus be located. Apply needle 1/2 inch deep or a little more to each point. The stimulus must be felt going down to the goiter.

Step Two: Apply needle to CV-22, 1 1/2″ deep, at an angle of 75 degrees. The stimulus will go up to the thyroid gland on both sides of the neck.

Step Three: Apply needle to LU-5, LU-7, BL-11, BL-12, and BL-13.

Step Four: Apply 5-7 direct moxa (green bean size) to CV-17.

• ***On the second and fifth days:***

Step One: Repeat steps one and two of the first day's treatment.

Step Two: Apply needle to BL-19, BL-20, BL-21, BL-23, and BL-25.

• *On the third and sixth days:*

Step One: Repeat steps one and two of the first day's treatment.

Step Two: Apply needle to ST-36, SP-6, BL-31, BL-32, BL-33, BL-34, CV-6, and CV-4.

Special Note: In the case of a simple goiter (that is, one affecting only the thyroid gland), **Steps One** and **Two** of the first day's treatment will suffice to cure the patient. In the case of an exophthalmic goiter, which is a toxic condition and affects other organs, e.g. the heart, eyes, or nerves, the more extensive treatment outlined above is necessary.

Prognosis: Thirty or more treatments are required.

Swelling of the Lymph Nodes of the Neck — Scrofula

Causes: The lymph nodes of the neck become infected by tuberculosis germs, which enter the lymph glands through the tonsils or through a decayed tooth. A weak body is particularly susceptible to this illness.

Symptoms: Groups of 10, and as many as 30 growths, some large and some small, appear on the neck of the patient. The small ones develop in size day by day, and in severe conditions the growths of scrofula go down under the arm, occasionally invading the lungs. If the patient is not treated, death will occur within a few years of the onset of the disease.

Treatment

• *Method I*

Step One: Apply needle to HT-3, TW-17, and XN-1 *(Pak Loh)*.

Step Two: Apply needle to the center of the scrofula lumps, withdraw the needle slightly, and then needle several corners of the lump.

Step Three: Apply indirect moxa with ginger to each scrofula lump, until the skin on each lump shows a reddish color from the heat of the moxa application.

Continue this treatment daily. The scrofula lumps will steadily decrease in size from day to day until the patient recovers completely.

• *Method II (Japanese Method)*

Step One: Take the left hand of the male or right hand of the female and hold open the hand with the four fingers close together and straight out.

Step Two: Measure across the fingers at the second joint of the pointing finger.

Step Three: Using the length derived from step two, measure from the bottom of the coccyx one such length up to a point on the sacrum.

Step Four: Apply from 10 to 20 direct moxa (peanut size) at the sacral point located in step three. The patient will feel the heat from the direct moxa reaching the abdomen and the two legs.

In mild conditions of scrofula, one treatment will suffice. In severe conditions, apply the treatment once every two weeks; after 3 or 4 treatments the patient should recover. In more severe cases, it may be necessary to give more treatments.

Not every patient will be able to stand direct moxa of peanut size. In these cases, for the first application knock the moxa off as soon as the patient feels that the heat is too much. During the second application, the patient will be able to tolerate greater heat from the moxa before reporting that the pain is too intense; the moxa will thus be allowed to burn closer to the skin. During the third application the moxa may be allowed to burn still nearer, and so on. However, do not count the partially burnt moxa as part of the treatment: The patient must have 10 to 20 moxa (peanut size) fully burnt down to the skin for the treatment to be fully effective.

- ***Method III***

Mix *Shyr Shiang* (musk) with moxa and apply this directly 5 to 7 times (red bean size) to HT-3. If the scrofula is on the left side of the neck, apply the direct moxa mixture to HT-3 on the left arm; if on the right side of the neck, apply the moxa to HT-3 on the right arm. For stronger stimulation and greater effect, the moxa may be applied to both arms.

In mild conditions, one treatment will be sufficient to bring about recovery. In severe conditions, renew the treatment every two weeks and continue for a few treatments until the patient recovers. Sexual relationships must be abandoned during this treatment, and for 120 days after treatment has been completed. If only one treatment was necessary, there must be no sexual relationship for 120 days after this one treatment, as the patient will be very weak as a consequence of his or her scrofula condition. *Do not use this treatment during menstruation or pregnancy.*

• ***Method IV***

Step One: Cut a piece of string the same length as the distance from the tip of the patient's middle finger (straight out) to the edge of the elbow (the olecranon process). Call this measurement *XY*.

Step Two: Take the string *XY* and place one end on GV-1 (point *Y*) and measure up the spine, marking the point on the patient's back at the other end of the string (point *X*).

Step Three: Cut another piece of string the same length as the distance from one corner of the lips to the other corner. Mark the center of this 2nd piece of string and call this point *X*. Call the 2nd string *PXQ*.

Step Four: Lay string *PXQ* on the patient's back so that both points *X* (on each string) coincide, and string *PXQ* is perpendicular to string *XY*.

Step Five: Apply 1 direct moxa (1/2″ diameter) once each to the end points, *P* and *Q*. If after application there is a blister, pierce the blister with a needle to withdraw the liquid, and cover with cotton wool.

After this treatment, the patient must not eat or drink cold fods or raw fruits. The patient will recover after only one such treatment, provided the directions are followed precisely.

• ***Method V (for mild conditions of scrofula)***

Step One: Measure string *XY* as in *Method IV* above.

Step Two: Place point *Y* at GV-1, and measure up the spine, marking point *X* at the tip of the string.

Step Three: Apply 5 direct moxa (yellow bean size) to point *X*, and 3 direct moxa (red bean size) on TW-17. If the scrofula is only on the left side, apply direct moxa to the TW-17 on the patient's left side and vice versa. If the scrofula has attacked both sides of the neck, apply direct moxa to TW-17 bilaterally.

If the patient's condition is mild and no older than one month, one application of this treatment will bring about a cure.

• *Method VI*

Step One: Place the patient's elbow on a table with the forearm vertical. Place a measuring rod at the tip of the elbow (point *C*) along the posterior surface of the forearm to the tip of the middle finger. Mark this distance on the stick, and call it point *A*. Take a second measurement, from the tip of the elbow to the tip of the ring finger of the same hand. Mark this distance on the stick and call it point *B*.

Step Two: Measure the distance between the patient's nipples, and cut a stick or a rod to this length. Place this second stick perpendicular to the first stick at point *B*, making a small cross with the two measuring sticks. The two ends of this second stick are called points *D*.

Step Three: Have the patient sit on a chair or stool with his or her back as straight as possible. Place the bottom of the crossed measuring sticks (point *C*) on the chair or stool seat with the cross itself vertically against the patient's back. Mark point *A* and both points *D* on the back.

Step Four: Apply 1 moxa (peanut size) on each of *A* and *D* points, starting the fire on all three moxa at the same time.

Assistant points: BL-20, HT-7, LI-11, GB-20, GB-21, LI-15, all with direct moxa.

Prescription I for Scrofula†	
Step One	Bring 3 pounds of vegetable oil to a boil in a copper pan.
Step Two	Add 20—30 live lizards, and boil until lizards are dissolved.
Step Three	Pour the oil into a jar, and allow to cool.
Step Four	Rub this oil on the scrofula and cover with a piece of cloth. Apply twice daily for an entire month.

†With this oil treatment, the moxa treatment may not be necessary, although use of both may be particularly helpful.

Prescription II for Scrofula	
Step One:	Feed *Jhu Sha* (Cinnabar) to 10 to 12 live white lizards for a few days. Keep the lizards in an earthenware jar during this time.
Step Two:	After this time, if the lizards' feces are the same color as the *Jhu Sha,* this indicates that their stomachs have been "purged," and that they are ready to be consumed.
Step Three:	Have the patient swallow one lizard alive* followed directly by a small cup of wine, for 7 to 10 days. In mild conditions, one lizard swallowed daily will suffice; in severe conditions it will be necessary to swallow one in the morning and one in the evening. Additional acupuncture or moxibustion may not be necessary.

*To swallow the lizard alive, hold it by its back legs. When opening the mouth, the patient should hold the lizard in such a position so that it will be anxious to run into the dark hold of the pharynx. The uvula will prevent the lizard from entering the trachea to the lungs. From the pharynx the lizard will run into the esophagus.

Special Note: It is common in cases of scrofula for several lumps to appear on the patient's neck. However, if there is only one lump, and this gradually grows bigger and bigger, it is more likely to be cancer. When a single growth the size and shape of half of an egg or half a potato appears first on one side of the neck and then on the other, like two pieces of board pressing the neck, the scrofula cannot be cured.

When there is a single growth on one side of the neck the size and shape of half a pigeon's egg, and it is found that the patient does not respond to acupuncture or moxibustion, to treatment with prescriptions I or II, or to a combination of several types of the treatments mentioned above, it is certain that the patient is not suffering from scrofula, but from cancer.

When a patient with scrofula becomes deaf, and his or her eyes seem to pop out of his or her head as though suffering from goiter, the patient will die, and no cure is possible with acupuncture.

Prognosis: Patients with scrofula of short duration or mild cases require one or two treatments. Patients with severe scrofula or who have had the scrofula for several years require 10 to 20 treatments for complete recovery.

Acute Tonsillitis

Causes: Germs in the throat; catching cold in the body.

Symptoms: The tonsils swell up, and the patient feels cold and has a temperature, pain in the pharynx, and difficulty swallowing. The tongue is coated, and the breath has an offensive odor. The pulse is rapid.

Treatment

• ***Treatment Method I***

Step One: Apply triangular needle to LU-11 and LI-1, obtaining a strong stimulus, and draw blood from both points.

Step Two: Apply needle to LI-4, TW-3, and LU-5.

Step Three: Apply needle to ST-6, GV-16, and CV-22.

Step Four: If the patient's condition is severe, apply a thick but *not* triangular needle to XF-8 *(Jin Jin/Yu Yeh),* KI-3, and BL-54, and draw out a few drops of blood from the veins at, or close to, the points.

• ***Treatment Method II***

Step One: Cut a piece of string the same length as the distance on the patient's hand from PC-7 to PC-9.

Step Two: Place one end of the string at the tip of the patient's nose and, keeping the string flat against the skin, run the string up the forehead along the centerline of the nose.

Step Three: At the tip of the string on the head, make a superficial incision along the skin not more than one half inch long with a scalpel. Cut downwards, in the direction of the forehead, and avoid cutting the flesh underneath. Express a few drops of blood.

• *Method III*

If there are one or two red spots close to GV-20, take a little nicotine from a smoker's pipe and apply on the red spots; the patient will then recover.

• *Method IV*

With the fingers, softly rub up and down about one inch on either side of the Adam's apple for about 20-30 seconds. This will bring out much phlegm from the throat, and will help ease the throat and facilitate recovery.

Prognosis: 2 to 3 treatments will suffice.

Inflammation of the Pharynx or Larynx

Pharyngitis

Causes: Catching cold or bad eating habits.

Symptoms: The pharynx is itchy and dry, and when swallowing there is some pain. There always seems to be a little phlegm in the pharynx and the patient desires to cough. The patient becomes hoarse and may even lose his or her voice temporarily. Except in mild conditions, there may be fever with feelings of coldness.

Laryngitis

Causes: Inflammation of the pharynx and catching cold; straining the vocal cords; irritating gases.

Symptoms: Itchiness in the larynx and pain if cold gets in; dry cough; hoarseness; difficulty in breathing. If the condition has been severe or present for a long time, the patient may lose the voice temporarily.

Treatment

• ***For Both Pharyngitis and Laryngitis***:

Step One: Apply needle to LI-4, LU-5, the point one division distal to LU-5 in the middle of the arm between two muscles, and to TW-3 and TW-2.

Step Two: Apply triangular needle to LU-11 and TW-1, and draw out a few drops of blood.

Step Three: Apply needle to KI-3. If the condition is severe, after applying needle to KI-3, find the vein close to KI-3 and draw out a few drops of blood by piercing the vein.

Inflammation with Dropsy in the Larynx

Causes: Inflammation of the patient's larynx from the second stage of syphilis; tuberculosis; diphtheria; very high fever; dropsy (edema) of the whole body.

Symptoms: The entire laryngial region is swollen, and continues to swell rapidly. The patient's breathing sounds like two cicadas, and the voice is very hoarse. Sometimes the patient will die within one or two hours.

Treatment

Step One: Apply triangular needle to LU-11 and TW-1, with strong stimulus, and draw out a few drops of blood.

Step Two: Apply needle to BL-54 and obtain a definite stimulus. Follow this with a triangular needle, piercing the vein close to BL-54 and drawing out a few drops of blood.

Step Three: Apply needle to KI-3 and obtain a stimulus. Follow this with a triangular needle, piercing the vein close to this point. Draw out a few drops of blood, as in the second step.

Step Four: Apply a long triangular needle to the throat region at the point where the larynx is swollen. Pierce a few spots in this area and draw out a few drops of blood or water.

Step Five: Apply needle to LI-4, TW-3, LU-5, one division under LU-5 in the middle of two muscles, GV-16, and CV-22. If the patient has a high fever, apply a triangular needle to PC-9 and TW-1, and draw out a few drops of blood.

Prognosis: Two or three treatments will bring about certain cure.

Diptheria

Causes: Infection by diptheria germs.

Symptoms: The patient's upper jaw, tonsils, and uvula are covered with the germs, and the region is coated with an ashen-white membrane. The patient has a high fever. Bronchitis often accompanies this condition and frequently is a cause of death.

Special Diagnosis: To differentiate between diptheria and tonsillitis, compare the color of the spots on the throat and the areas in which they appear. In the case of tonsillitis, the white spots on the throat are somewhat yellowish in color; in diptheria, the color is white and ashen. In tonsillitis, only the tonsil region is white and yellow. In diptheria, the white and ashen color is found not only on the tonsils, but on the upper jaw as well; it may even extend to, and beyond, the uvula.

Treatment

Step One: Apply needle to LI-4, TW-3, and LU-5, and to the point one division below LU-5 in the middle of two muscles.

Step Two: Apply triangular needle to LU-11 and TW-1. First obtain a strong stimulus, and then draw out a few drops of blood from both of these points.

Step Three: Apply needle to GV-14, GV-16, ST-6, and CV-22.

Step Four: Apply triangular needle to XF-8 *(Jin Jin/Yu Yeh)* and draw out a few drops of blood. If the patient is unconscious, use an instrument to hold the tongue so that the triangular needle can reach the point under the tongue.

Prognosis: In the early stages of diptheria, three or four treatments will bring about recovery. In the advanced stages, it is almost impossible to save the patient.

Prescription I for Diptheria	
Step One	Take the skin off of one or two large pieces of garlic and pound the garlic into mush.
Step Two	Apply the garlic to LI-5 and allow the skin to swell up until a blister forms. This process may be painful, but is essential.
Step Three	Pierce the blister with a needle and extract all the fluid within it.

Prescription II for Diptheria
Blow *Wu P'ei Tzu Powder* (Galla Rhi Chinensis et Potaninii) twice daily into the region of the throat affected by the diptheria. This will help recovery.

Carbuncle in the Throat

Causes: Excessive consumption of "overheating" foods or alcoholic beverages.

Symptoms: Inflammation of the throat, with swelling, pain, and redness on the neck below the jaw. In severe conditions, the carbuncle may contain pus, and may pierce the skin either on the outside of the neck or on the inside of the throat.

Treatment

Step One: Apply needle to LI-4 and LI-11.

Step Two: Apply a triangular needle to LU-11 and TW-1. Obtain a strong stimulus and draw out a few drops of blood.

Step Three: Apply needle to SP-10, BL-54, GB-20, ST-6, and CV-22.

Step Four: If a little pain goes up to the ear following the third step, apply needle to GB-2.

Step Five: If there is no pus inside of the carbuncle, apply indirect moxa with ginger to the region of the swelling on the outside of the neck. Then saturate a piece of cotton wool in Rivenal water and apply several times daily, also to the outside of the neck.

Step Six: If pus comes through the skin at the neck, use white ointment or Red Jade ointment. If the pus is inside, whether or not it pierces the skin, gargle frequently with boric acid solution, holding the solution in the mouth for some time.

Step Seven: If the patient has no fever, whether or not there is pus, apply 7 direct moxa (red bean size) on LI-11 of both arms. This will be a great help toward recovery. If the condition is severe and direct moxa on LI-11 does not help, apply 5 direct moxa (red bean size) to SP-10. The result of this additional treatment will be satisfactory. If the patient suffers from constipation, a laxative should be taken to keep the bowels moving daily.

Prognosis: In the early stages of the disease, three treatments will suffice. If there has been pus on either the inside or the outside, 7 to 10 treatments will be necessary. If the openings are on both sides of the neck, it may be difficult for acupuncture to be of help.

Acute Bronchitis
— Coughing —

Causes: Catching cold; catarrh of the nose.

Symptoms: A little cough with phlegm; hoarseness of the voice; tiredness of the whole body; pain in the joints. Fever will generally not be present in mild conditions. In severe conditions, however, a fever of 38 °C to 39 °C may be expected.

Treatment

Step One: Apply needle to LI-4 and LU-7.

Step Two: Apply needle to GV-14, BL-12, and BL-13. If there is no fever, follow with indirect moxa on these points, applying the heat until the skin around the points is red.

Step Three: If there is a little pain in the chest after applying steps one and two, apply needle to LU-9.

Step Four: If there is an itching sensation in the throat, apply needle to CV-22 and LU-5.

Step Five: If there is much phlegm, apply needle to ST-40, leaving the needle in the point for at least 15 minutes after obtaining the stimulus.

Step Six: If there is fever, apply needle to LI-11 and BL-54.

Step Seven: If the cough is very dry, apply triangular needle to LU-11 and draw out a few drops of blood.

Prognosis: In mild conditions, three treatments will be necessary. In severe conditions, about seven treatments will be required.

Prescription I for Dry Cough or Whooping Cough		
Herb		Quantity
Chinese	Pharmaceutical Name	
蚌花	*Flos Magnolia Officinalis*	2-3 oz
紅棗	*Fructus Zizyphi Jujubae*	10-15 pcs

Boil the above ingredients with three bowls of water until one bowl of water remains. Drink in one dose.

Prescription II for Dry Cough or Whooping Cough		
Herb		Quantity
Chinese	Pharmaceutical Name	
枇杷葉	*Folium Eriobotryae*	1/2 oz
密棗	*Fructus Zizyphi (preserved)*	7 pcs
	Fresh duck egg with bluish shell	1

Place the above ingredients in three bowls of water and boil until the duck egg is hardboiled. After the egg is hardboiled, remove the shell and return the egg to the decoction. Continue boiling until the liquid is reduced to one bowl. Give this to the patient to drink. This will greatly help the condition.

Note: *Gwa Sha* on the upper back and along the ribs may also be useful in this condition.

Pneumonia with Catarrh

Causes: High fever; bronchitis; inflammation of the larynx.

Symptoms: Expectoration of liquid from the lungs; sudden high fever with severe cough and vomiting; poor appetite; fast pulse; rapid breathing; cold hands and feet. The muscles become tinged with blue.

Treatment

Step One: Apply needle to LI-4, LU-7, LU-9, LU-5, and LI-11.

Step Two: Apply needle to GV-14, GV-13, BL-12, and BL-13.

Step Three: Apply needle to BL-54.

Step Four: Apply triangular needle to LU-11 and draw out a few drops of blood. If there is much phlegm, apply needle to ST-40 to a depth of 2 to 3 inches in adults, 1 to 1 1/2 inches in children.

Prognosis: First stages are easily cured in one to three treatments. Severe conditions indicate a serious disease, and will require many treatments. In these cases, acupuncture can be a great help.

Tuberculosis of the Lungs

Causes: Tuberculosis germs entering the lungs; lack of fresh air and sunshine. People who fall into the following categories are most susceptible to contracting the disease:

- Those between 18 and 30 years of age;
- Those with anemia or diabetes;
- Women post-partum;
- Those who have been depressed for a long time;
- Those who are in close contact with others who have tuberculosis;
- Those whose diet is inadequate;
- Those who are thin and narrow-chested, with a long neck and narrow face.

Symptoms: In the beginning, the patient has a poor appetite and suffers from anemia and a mild temperature. The patient feels a numb sensation when his or her chest is touched, as if there is a piece of paper placed between your fingers and the patient's skin. Compared with the entire chest, the affected side of the chest seems smaller. When the patient inhales and exhales, there appears to be less movement on the affected side. The patient does not feel pain in the lungs, even when the lungs have become ulcerated. With most tuberculosis patients there is coughing, although coughing may be insignificant or absent in some cases. In the beginning, unless there are holes in the lungs, very little phlegm is expectorated. This phlegm often contains small amounts of blood, although there are those who do not bring up blood at all.

The fever at the beginning stages is relatively low, 37.2 ° to 38 °C. In the last stages of tuberculosis, the fever will be normal in the mornings and rise to 39 ° or 40 °C in the afternoon. Others have a high fever in the morning which regularly drops in the afternoon. If the illness advances very slowly, there will be only a slight fever. If there is a wide fluctuation in the patient's fever between the morning and afternoon, this is a sign of a very serious condition.

The pulse of the tuberculosis patient is fast and weak. The tuberculosis patient also suffers from night sweating which, if left unchecked, may cause the patient to loose weight rapidly (a common symptom in tuberculosis patients) and possibly bring on death. The skin of the tuberculosis patient is dry and has a pale ashen color, with some flushing of the face near the cheekbone. In the last stages, most tuberculosis patients contract dropsy in some parts of the body or over the whole body. Sometimes the dropsy is in the feet or hands alone.

Special Note: Before applying acupuncture, take the patient's temperature and keep a record of his or her pulse rates. Although there might not be other evidence of progress, a steady, day by day drop in temperature and slowing of the pulse rate indicate that the disease is being arrested and that the patient is on the road to recovery. When applying the needle, the acupuncturist must cover his or her mouth and nose.

Treatment

Step One: Apply needle to LI-4, LU-7, and LU-5.

Step Two: Apply needle to GV-14, BL-12, and BL-13.

Step Three: Apply indirect moxa with ginger to all points of the second step.

Step Four: If there is an itch in the throat, apply needle to CV-22.

Step Five: If there is much phlegm being brought up, apply needle to ST-40. The needle should go in two to three inches, according to the size of the patient.

Step Six: If there is coughing with blood, apply needle to BL-18.

Step Seven: If there is night sweating, apply needle to HT-6 and KI-8. If the night sweating does not cease after using these points, apply 3 direct moxa (green bean size) to HT-6 and KI-8.

Step Eight: If the patient suffers from lack of appetite, apply needle to PC-6, ST-36, and CV-12. After applying the needle to CV-12, apply indirect moxa with ginger to that point.

Step Nine: If patient pants, apply needle to CV-6 and apply indirect moxa with ginger to CV-17.

Step Ten: If after a few treatments the fever has not been lowered, apply needle to KI-1, ST-36, and GV-4.

Step Eleven: If the patient coughs a great deal, apply needle to GV-13, GV-12, and ST-18.

Step Twelve: If the patient feels as though something were pressing on his or her chest, causing labored breathing, apply needle to LU-9, LU-1, and LV-14.

This treatment must be continued for seven to ten days. If after this period the patient's temperature has returned to normal, apply direct moxa as follows:

- Five direct moxa (green bean size) on GV-14 daily for three days
- Five direct moxa (green bean size) on BL-12 daily the next three days
- Five direct moxa (green bean size) on BL-13 daily the next three days

If the patient has been able to endure the pain, after this nine-day treatment with direct moxa apply 3 direct moxa (green bean size) on GV-14, BL-12, and BL-13 daily. Continue with this treatment for five to seven days. It is not necessary to needle these points during the moxa treatment. However, following this period, needle the points every day until the patient has fully recovered. In order not to pierce the burnt skin with the needle on these three points, move the skin away from the area of the moxa burn with the forefinger, using the middle finger to press the skin down for puncturing.

If, after the above treatments, the patient does not recover, apply 5 direct moxa (green bean size) to BL-15 for 5 days. Then apply 7 direct moxa (red bean size) to ST-36 daily for 10 days. If the patient's kidneys are weak and "empty," in addition to the above treatments, apply 5 direct moxa (red bean size) to BL-23 daily, for 5 to 7 days.

Special Note: In all cases of tuberculosis, do not use direct moxa for the first 7 to 10 days. Only when the temperature has returned to normal may direct moxa be used. However, during this time indirect moxa may be used with the needle as instructed. Be extremely cautious in the use of direct moxa in patients under the age of 25, even after the seven to ten day period. In these cases, continue with needles and indirect moxa for several days longer than usual before considering treatment with direct moxa, even if the temperature has returned to normal.

For middle-aged and older patients, it will be necessary to apply direct moxa as indicated even before the patient's temperature has returned to normal.

Prognosis: In the early stages, prompt treatment will cure this disease easily and speedily. If the patient's body is naturally strong, recovery will be rapid and without complications. Weak patients will be less responsive to treatment.

Young patients commonly contract the acute form of tuberculosis, which is more difficult to cure. In elderly patients, the tuberculosis will most likely be chronic, and will thus be more responsive to treatment. Persons who have no financial worries, who are not required to work for a living, who have no heavy sorrows, are not burdened with heavy responsibilities, are not bad tempered or easily irritated, and who have gentle dispositions and good appetites respond to treatment far more easily than those with these traits. If the patient suffers from inflammation in the pharynx or larynx or from tuberculosis of the intestines, the condition will be more difficult to cure. If the patient suffers from pleurisy and pneumothorax (rupture of the lung cavity), effecting a cure will be difficult.

In the early stages, about 30 treatments will bring about recovery. In the middle stages, about two to three months will bring about recovery. In the advanced stages, the treatment may assist in prolonging the patient's life, but there is no certainty of recovery.

Dropsy in the Lungs

Causes: Pneumonia; inflammation of the kidneys due to impaired function of water excretion, which causes water to remain in the tissues and lungs; advanced stages of some "overcooling" illness (e.g., dropsy). Liquid passes from the blood vessels of the lungs into the lung tissue. This illness always occurs suddenly at night.

Symptoms: Chest discomfort, and possibly some chest pain; difficulty in breathing, accompanied by a short and quick cough with much phlegm; wheezing. The patient has a pale face, and sweats all over the face and body. The pulse and heart are weak. Sometimes the patient will die in a few hours. If the crisis stage has passed, in 12 to 24 hours the patient will get better and the disease will change into a chronic condition. In the chronic condition, the water will accumulate in all parts of the body, producing edema.

Treatment

Step One: Apply needle to LI-4, LU-7, and LU-9.

Step Two: Apply needle to GV-14, BL-12, BL-13, and BL-23.

Step Three: Apply needle to LU-1, CV-4, and SP-9.

• *Additional Treatment*: Look at the region of the thoracic vertebrae between the 1st and the 12th vertebrae. If there are any red or black spots on the skin exactly over the region of the vertebrae, take a triangular needle and pierce the spot. If there is more than one spot in the region, pierce one or two and express a few drops of blood.

Prognosis: This is a very serious illness. Breathing becomes increasingly difficult and shorter, the pulse gets weaker and weaker, the patient gradually loses consciousness, ceases to breathe, and finally dies. If this illness is discovered early and acupuncture treatment is applied immediately, it will be easy for the patient to recover. In acute conditions, about 10 treatments are necessary. About 20 treatments are required in chronic conditions.

Hemoptysis

Causes: In some young patients, blood is suddenly expectorated from the lungs. In many cases, this is indicative of "overheated" lungs, and no other disease will be found. In other cases, this is caused by tuberculosis in the lungs, pneumonia, heart disease, or from decay and breaking of the lining of the larynx or the bronchus and the resulting hemorrhage. In women, the menses sometimes cease and blood comes out from the lungs, stomach or nose.

Symptoms: When coughing, phlegm mixed with blood is expectorated. In acute conditions, much blood is expectorated in a short time. If the blood vessels have burst there will be a lot of blood coming out; this is very serious.

Treatment

Step One: Apply needle to LI-4, LU-7, and LU-5.

Step Two: Apply needle to ST-36.

Step Three: Apply needle to GV-14, BL-12, and BL-13.

Step Four: Apply needle to BL-18, and obtain only a light stimulus, retaining the needle in the point to maintain the light stimulus for a few seconds.

Step Five: If the patient feels that there is something pressing on or gripping his or her chest, apply needle to LU-9.

Step Six: If the patient feels an itchy sensation in the throat, apply needle to CV-22.

Step Seven: If the patient feels very tired, tense, or tight in the muscles of the back, apply needle to BL-38.

Prognosis: In mild conditions one or two treatments will suffice. In severe conditions 7 to 10 treatments will be necessary.

Prescription I for Hemoptysis		
Herb		Quantity
Chinese	Pharmaceutical Name	
牛七	*Radix Achyranthes*	5-10 pcs

Boil these in a bowl of water for two to three minutes. Allow to cool a little and have the patient drink this concoction while it is still warm.

Prescription II for Hemoptysis		
Herb		Quantity
Chinese	Pharmaceutical Name	
連翹	*Ramulus Nelumbinis Nuciferae*	1 lb

The common English name for *Lian Gen* is Lotus Root. Grind the lotus root and squeeze the juice from it. Drink the expressed juice. The bleeding will stop immediately.

Asthma

Causes: This illness is caused by cramp in the bronchus, resulting in great difficulty breathing. Asthma is easily affected by sudden changes in weather, such as temperature and humidity fluctuations.

Symptoms: The condition comes on very suddenly, usually in the evening. The patient has difficulty breathing, pants, and cannot sleep lying down, preferring to sit with his or her head resting down in front. The pulse is narrow, fast, and small. When the asthmatic attack is approaching, the patient sweats a great deal. It is only during the periods of an attack of asthma that the patient shows the above symptoms. In the intervening periods, the patient is normal.

Treatment

Step One: Apply needle to LI-4 and LU-7.

Step Two: Apply needle to GV-14, BL-12, and BL-13.

Step Three: Apply indirect moxa with ginger to all points of step two until the skin changes to a reddish color.

Step Four: Apply needle to GV-22, angling the needle 75° and inserting it to a depth of 1/2 inch.

Step Five: Apply needle to ST-40, to a depth of 3 inches. After obtaining the stimulus, let the needle remain in the point for half an hour without endeavoring to obtain any further stimulus.

Step Six: Apply 7 direct moxa (green bean size) to GV-10. After these 6 steps, the panting should cease, and breathing should be back to normal.

Step Seven: If the patient has much phlegm in his or her lungs, apply needle to LU-5.

Step Eight: If the patient's heart is too weak, apply the needle to a point one eye division on both sides of the point below the 4th cervical vertebrae; also apply 5 moxa (green bean size) on CV-14.

Step Nine: If the patient's kidneys are very weak (sometimes the asthma is caused by weakness in the kidneys) apply 5 direct moxa (green bean size) to BL-23. If the spleen and stomach are very weak, apply 5 direct moxa (green bean size) to
BL-20, CV-12, ST-36, and LV-13.

Step Ten: If there is a wheezing sound from the bronchus when the patient breathes, apply 5 direct moxa (green bean size) to CV-22 or CV-17.

Step Eleven: If the patient's lungs are very weak and/or manifest an "overcooling" condition, after a few daily treatments apply 5 direct moxa (green bean size) to GV-14, BL-12, and BL-13. Continue the direct moxa treatment daily for a few days.

Assistant Points: LV-14, LI-16, CV-23, GV-9, CV-6.

Prognosis: Medicine will merely relieve an attack of asthma, but acupuncture treatment can actually cure the condition. In acute or mild conditions, about 7 treatments will cure the patient completely. In severe or chronic conditions, about 20 to 30 treatments will be required to effect a complete cure, thus preventing the return of further attacks.

Special Note: Patients who are subject to attacks in the autumn and winter months are more easily cured then those who are subject to attacks all year round. The asthmatic should avoid cold foods and drinks, as these help to bring on the attacks.

Prescription I for Asthma	
Step One	Obtain a live frog.
Step Two	Fill the frog's mouth with whole peppercorns, and bind its mouth and legs with thread.
Step Three	Wrap the live frog in soft wet clay and place it on a charcoal stove, allowing it to burn until the clay dries up and there is no more smoke. The frog and pepper should be completely charred.
Step Four	Allow the frog to cool.
Step Five	Grind the frog into a fine powder.
Step Six	Place 1/7 oz. of this powder in 1-2 T. of wine.
Step Seven	Have the patient drink one such decoction each day until he or she recovers.

Prescription II for Asthma	
Step One	Place 1/2 ounce of *Herba Ephedrae* and 1/7 ounce of *Radix Glycyrrhizae* in two cups of water.
Step Two	Bring to a boil and cook until less than one cup of liquid remains. Drink when warm.
Step Three	Repeat for three days. The asthma will be completely better.

Palpitation of the Heart

Causes: Too much mental activity; hysteria; excessive sexual intercourse; anemia.

Symptoms: Even without placing the hand over the heart, the patient can feel his or her heart palpitating. The patient feels a little pressure on his or her chest and some difficulty breathing. Even doing work without physical exertion, such as walking up and down stairs, the patient feels palpitations.

Treament

- ***Treatment I for Heart Palpitations***

Step One: Apply needle to PC-6, PC-5, HT-5, and HT-7.

Step Two: Apply needle to GB-20, BL-10, GV-14, and BL-15, obtaining light stimulus from all points.

Step Three: Apply 5 direct moxa (green bean size) to GV-11.

- ***Treatment II for Heart Palpitations***

Needle the points one division bilaterally from under the fourth and fifth cervical vertebrae to a depth of one inch. The palpitations will cease as soon as the stimulus is felt.

Prognosis: In mild conditions, 5 treatments are necessary. In chronic and severe conditions, 10 treatments are required.

Note: Before treating, balance the heart.

Angina Pectoris

Causes: Hardening and narrowing of the wall of the coronary arteries; inflammation of the muscles of the heart; syphilis. This disease is more common among gentle folk and seldom occurs in laborers. It is usually contracted between 40 and 70 years of age, and is more common in men than in women.

Symptoms: There are 3 types of Angina Pectoris: *True Angina Pectoris, Angina Pectoris of the Nerves,* and *Angina Pectoris of the Blood Vessels.*

True Angina Pectoris primarily affects the elderly. Although attacks of angina are often sudden and unexpected, usually the attack is preceded by feelings of pressure over the heart and general heart discomfort, perspiration over the entire body, and depression. When the angina develops, the patient suddenly feels very severe, almost unendurable pains in the heart under the sternum, as if death is imminent. There may be shortness of breath, cold arms and legs, and cold sweat.

Angina Pectoris of the Nerves attacks young people. The symptoms are the same as in true angina pectoris, though less severe, and the patient does not die easily from it. However, with frequent attacks, the patient's heart will be greatly weakened, and by the time the patient reaches middle age, a true case of angina pectoris will have developed.

Angina Pectoris of the Blood Vessels occurs in cold weather, in patients who are often chilled and who lack nourishing food, whose arms and legs become stiff and turn white with cold. The condition of the heart resembles that of a patient suffering from angina pectoris. The pumping action of the heart steadily weakens as it becomes colder and colder, finally ending in death.

Treatment

Step One: Apply needle to PC-6, PC-5, HT-7, HT-5, HT-4, and HT-8.

Step Two: Apply needle to SP-1, ST-36, and BL-15.

Step Three: Apply green bean size direct moxa to PC-5. In mild conditions, apply 7 moxa. In severe conditions, apply 14 moxa.

Step Four: In very severe conditions, after the above mentioned steps have been taken, apply 7 direct moxa 1/2 rice grain size) to *Tu Yin* (under the second toe, at the center of the second crease). If the condition is not very severe, it would be better to wait for the second day to apply this step.

Step Five: Apply 5 direct moxa (green bean size) to CV-14. Although this step is very effective, if the preceding steps are sufficiently effective, it would be appropriate to use this step on the 3rd day of treatment only. In very serious cases, however, apply this step beginning on the first day.

• *Special Treatment for Angina Pectoris*

If the acupuncturist is confronted with a patient just as the attack of angina pectoris is occurring, there may be insufficient time to apply all the steps of the treatment outlined above; swift action may be necessary in order to save the patient's life. In this case, apply needle to PC-5, HT-7, and HT-4 as quickly as possible and obtain a stimulus from each point. The patient will obtain some comfort from this immediate treatment. The acupuncturist should at once apply 14 direct moxa (red bean size) to PC-5 bilaterally. After this treatment, the patient will feel much more comfortable. Finally, apply 7 direct moxa (green bean size) to XT-1 *(Tu Yin),* burning the moxa on both feet. This treatment will save the patient.

Prognosis: Angina patients can definitely be cured by acupuncture. Mild conditions require 5 to 7 treatments; severe conditions about 20 treatments. Sudden severe attacks cannot be saved without immediate treatment by acupuncture.

Inflammation of the Mammary Gland

Causes: A woman, usually a strong woman, with a first birth produces too much milk. The infant can not consume all of the milk and milk remains in the breast. The breast swells, and milk stagnates in the nipple, blocking the passage.

Symptoms: The breast is swollen, hot, hard and red, with pain that radiates to the center of the chest. If, when the nipple is blocked, the condition is not treated in time, the entire breast may become a ulcerated, oozing puss. This is difficult to cure.

Treatment

Step One: Needle LI-4 and PC-6.

Step Two: Use one half-rice size direct moxa at SI-1.

Step Three: Needle ST-18, manipulating the needle for about ten seconds until the stimulation goes throughout the breast.

Step Four: Needle ST-16.

Step Five: Apply seven green bean size direct moxa to CV-17.

Step Six: Use indirect moxa with ginger on the hardest area of the breast three times, the area will then soften.

Auxilary Treatment: Use a breast pump to remove the stagnant milk. Even when fresh milk begins to flow, continue until all the milk has been expressed.

Prescription: Clean and pound to a paste an entire dandelion plant. Boil the paste in one cup of cooking wine until 1/2 a cup remains. The patient should drink the wine, saving the dregs to use as a plaster for the breast.

Special Note: In cases where it is not simply inflammation of the mammary gland, but where there is an actual carbuncle on the breast, use the same treatment eliminating step five (moxa at CV-17). Instead, use ten red bean size moxa at LI-11 and needle SP-10 and BL-54. Apply white ointment to the carbuncle.

Prognosis: Three to five treatments should be sufficient.

Cancer of the Breast in the Initial Stages

Causes: A period of great sorrow and grief with excessive crying; desperation under great vicissitudes; a long period of worry and trouble; eating foods with artificial coloring; excessive breathing of smoke; unnatural growth of tissue in the body which has not been successfully destroyed by the body's natural defenses. This growth of unnatural tissue increases rapidly in size, forms a small lump, and joins with the normal tissue around it, forming a tumor.

Symptoms: The cancerous growth in the breast is at first the size of a soybean, and gradually grows bigger and bigger. The patient begins to feel a little pain in the region as the growth enlarges. If it grows to the size of an egg when you touch it, it will feel fixed inside. After some time (perhaps 6 months to a year) the pain increases and becomes severe, radiating to other parts of the chest above and below the armpit. As the tumor grows larger, rounder, and harder, the skin of the chest or breast becomes very shiny, and very small red veins will become visible. These veins may even bleed through the skin. Soon, the skin will break open, exuding offensive and purulent fluid mixed with blood. This ulceration finally forms a crater, which may even get infected with maggots. In this condition, although there may be no pain, there will be itching. At this point the patient is in the final stages of breast cancer, which will now be incurable.

In the early stage, that is, when the lump of the cancer in the breast can be moved with the fingers (i.e., before it becomes fixed) the cancer can be successfully treated by acupuncture. When the cancer has grown larger and is fixed inside so that you cannot move the lump away from its position, it is much more difficult to cure, and treatment by acupuncture may fail. However, in some cases acupuncture treatment is successful even though the cancer is so far advanced. If a biopsy has been performed by a medical doctor, it is best to avoid treating the patient with acupuncture, since the biopsy may stimulate additional cancerous growths by allowing the cancer cells to spread throughout the body.

Treatment

Step One: Apply needle to LU-9, PC-6, and LI-4, and apply 1 direct moxa (1/2 rice grain size) to SI-1.

Step Two: Apply needle to GB-21 penetrating 1 1/2 inch deep. Send the stimulus down the chest. Before taking this step, feel the pulse to ascertain the condition of the heart. *If the patient suffers from heart palpitations, angina pectoris, or even weakness of the heart, GB-21 is not to be used.*

Step Three: Apply needle to ST-16 and ST-18, and 7 direct moxa (red bean size) to CV-17.

Step Four: Apply indirect moxa with ginger to the cancerous lump. If the cancer has reached the second stage, that is, if it is fixed in its position, rather than applying indirect moxa to the lump, use a long, thick needle and apply it into the lump. Burn 3 balls of moxa the size of pigeon's eggs on the handle of the needle, one after the other.

Assistant Points: PC-7, LU-5, ST-36, BL-54, GB-44.

Prognosis: In the first stage, which is easy to cure, 3 to 7 treatments should suffice. In the second stage, it is very difficult to cure, though in some cases acupuncture is effective: use as many treatments as the patient requires to obtain a cure. In the third or last stage, no cure is possible.

Intercostal Neuralgia

Causes: Any disease in the rib bones or in the vertebrae, or neuralgia of the vertebrae. Chinese doctors say that another cause of pain in the ribs is constant anger.

Symptoms: Pain in the nerves between any of the ribs. The pain is semicircular. If this pain continues for a long period it will spread to other parts of the body, including the chest and back. Sometimes the pain is so severe that it is painful to cough and even to breathe. This illness invariably starts in the left side between the 5th and 9th ribs.

Treatment

Step One: Apply needle to TW-6 and GB-34 on both sides.

Step Two: Apply needle to LV-14 on the affected side. If the condition is mild, these two steps will be sufficient to effect a cure.

Step Three: After this treatment, if there is some pain under or close to the chest, apply needle to ST-18. If there is some place on the ribs where there is still some pain, apply a needle followed by indirect moxa with an instrument or ginger to that spot.

Step Four: If there is pain in the upper part of the back, apply needle to BL-13. If there is some pain in the middle part of the back, apply needle to BL-18.

Step Five: If the condition constitutes an ''overcooling'' condition, and after applying the needle there still remains a little pain, apply indirect moxa to BL-18 or to the spot or spots that are painful. If indirect moxa does not suffice and still some pain remains, apply 3 direct moxa (green bean size) to BL-18 and/or to the painful places.

Step Six: If this is an "overheating" condition, use the needle in place of the points mentioned above for steps 1-4 and do not use moxa at all. For "overheating" conditions, also apply needle to GB-21, 1/2 inch deep, to the side that is affected. *If the heart is weak, or if there is angina pectoris or the patient suffers from palpitations, substitute HT-8 for GB-21.*

Prognosis: Two or three treatments will suffice even in severe conditions. In mild conditions, 1 treatment may suffice.

Inflammation of the Esophagus

Causes: Consumption of too many strong tasting foods (e.g., mustard, red chili, curry, etc.); swallowing articles like pins, bits of pencil, etc.; consuming food or drink that is too hot; over-indulgence in wine; excessive smoking.

Symptoms: In mild conditions, there is only discomfort when swallowing or drinking food. In severe conditions, there is pain in the esophagus and under the chest bone when swallowing. This develops into a condition in which the patient cannot swallow because of the pain. In very severe conditions, the food swallowed is brought up again, and the patient may even vomit out a little pus. Even in severe conditions, only the esophagus is affected and the patient can talk and can do everything else normally.

Treatment

Step One: Apply needle to LI-4, PC-6, and LU-9.

Step Two: Apply needle to GB-21 and penetrate 1 1/2 inches (the stimulus should go down to the chest). *Be careful not to use the needle in this point if the patient suffers from weakness of the heart, palpitations, or angina pectoris.*

Step Three: Apply needle to CV-22 at a 75 degree slant and penetrate 1 1/2 to 1 3/4 inches. The stimulus must reach the stomach. Continue with 5 direct moxa (green bean size) to CV-22.

Step Four: Apply needle to CV-12 and CV-13.

Step Five: Apply indirect moxa with ginger to CV-17 and CV-16.

Step Six: If the condition is severe or chronic, apply 7 direct moxa (½ rice grain size) to Jung Kuei and 7 green bean size to BL-17. One can also apply 7 direct moxa on CV-17 and CV-16 (green bean size), one point on each day.

Prognosis: In mild conditions, 1 or 2 treatments are necessary. In severe or chronic cases, 7 treatments are necessary.

Stenosis of the Esophagus

Causes: Growth, tumor, or cancer in the esophagus; swelling of the heart; some illness in the diaphragm; cramp of the esophagus.

Symptoms: In the early stages the patient finds it difficult to swallow food, and can only take liquids. Gradually the esophagus becomes narrower and the patient is unable even to drink liquids. The patient is hungry, tired, and thin, and his or her face is pale. Eventually death by starvation occurs.

Treatment

Step One: Apply needle to LI-4, LU-7, and LU-9.

Step Two: Apply needle to ST-36 and ST-44.

Step Three: Apply needle to GB-21, penetrating 1 1/2 inches. The stimulus should go down the chest. *Omit this step if the patient suffers from any diseases of the heart.*

Step Four: Apply needle to CV-22 at a 75 degree angle and penetrate 1 1/2 to 1 3/4 inches. The stimulus should go down to the stomach.

Step Five: Apply needle to CV-13 and CV-12.

Step Six: Apply indirect moxa with ginger, or direct moxa, to CV-16 and CV-17.

Step Seven: Needle BL-15 and BL-17, and continue with indirect moxa with ginger or instrument to these points.

Prognosis: In the first stage, the patient is easily cured and requires only 5 to 7 treatments. If the esophagus has become completely closed up, a cure will be impossible.

Neurosis, Gastritis, or Stomach Cramps

Causes: Overproduction of digestive juices, stomach ulcer, stomach tumor, disharmonies in the organs surrounding the stomach (liver, pancreas, intestines), poisioning, lead or mercury poisioning, chronic malaria, rheumatism, spinal TB, spinal inflammation, neurotic stomachache, asthenia. This condition is associated with weak, pale, overcooling patients and may be associated with conditions evidenced by ovarian turmors, uterine disorders, amenorehea, or nocturnal loss of semen.

Symptoms: In the early stages there is a feeling of heavy oppression in the stomach area and nausea. The ache begins in the upper abdomen, then moves to the left side of the body. There can be severe pain under the chest, and the attack can last from several minutes to several hours. The patient will be pale and will bend forward in response to the pain. The pain may be relieved by pressure.

Special Diagnosis: When the patient's pain is relieved by pressure it is an overcooling condition. Overheating patients will refuse pressure. If the attack commences after the patient has eaten a full meal, a stomach carbuncle is indicated. If the pain arrives when the patient is hungry, the stomach membrane has been damaged from excess gastric juices irritating the area. An excess of gastric juices is accompanied by a sour taste in the mouth.

Neurosis, Gastritis, or Stomach Cramps		
Principal Points	Assistant Points	Auxiliary Points
PC-6, ST-36 CV-12	ST-44, SP-4 CV-13, CV-10, CV-8, CV-6	CV-14, KI-16 BL-20, BL-21, BL-22, CV-11

Treatment

Step One: Needle PC-6 and ST-36.

Step Two: Needle CV-12. If the patient is not overheating, use indirect moxa. In light cases, this will be sufficient to cure the condition.

Step Three: If pain remains above CV-12, needle CV-12 and CV-14.

Step Four: If pain remains under CV-12, needle CV-10 and CV-11.

Step Five: If pain that reaches to the umbilicus remains, needle CV-6. Fill the umbilicus with salt and apply green bean size moxa ten times.

Step Six: If pain remains that reaches to the back, needle BL-20 and BL-21.

Step Seven: If the pain is still not completely relieved, apply five direct moxa, green been size, to CV-12. However, in the case of overheating patients use needles at ST-44 and SP-4 instead.

Step Eight: In the case of a surfeit of gastric juices, or pain that accompanies hunger, apply direct moxa, red bean size, to GB-34a. Do not moxa ST-36, as this will increase the production of gastric juices.

Prognosis: Light cases will be cured in one or two treatments; chronic cases require approximately ten treatments.

Acute Inflammation of the Stomach — Vomiting —

Causes: This common illness is caused by eating undigestible foods, overeating, or eating stale food or overripe fruit. These irritate the mucus membrane of the stomach and cause the patient to loose his or her appetite and to vomit. In children, this condition is accompanied by diarrhea.

Symptoms: At first, the patient has no appetite, and feels discomfort in the abdomen. This will be followed by headache, eructation, and vomiting, first of food and then of phlegm and gastric juices. Sometimes there is fever and the patient feels cold.

Treatment

Step One: Apply needle to PC-6.

Step Two: Apply needle to ST-36a.

Step Three: Apply needle to CV-12, and then apply indirect moxa with ginger or instrument to the two points of the second and third steps.

Step Four: If the patient also suffers from diarrhea, apply needle to ST-25, CV-6, and CV-4, and then apply indirect moxa with ginger or instrument to these 3 points. If the patient also has fever and feels cold, apply needle to LI-4, GB-20, GV-14, and BL-12.

In addition to the above treatment, use **Prescription V** for **Influenza.**

Prognosis: One or two treatments should suffice.

Vomiting Due to Upset Nerves of the Stomach

Causes: Motion sickness; meningitis; tuberculosis in the spinal cord; something directly touching and thus irritating the stomach from the inside or outside; something irritating the throat or the peritoneum; pregnancy; any gynecological disorder.

Nervous vomiting appears in four distinct symptom patterns:

Symptom Pattern A: In this condition, vomiting is easily induced in the patient, and recurs frequently, usually following a meal. The period of vomiting is usually of short duration, and is preceded by eructation.

Symptom Pattern B: In this condition, dry vomiting comes on suddenly. The patient's arms and legs are cold and the pulse can hardly be felt. This condition is quite serious, and can lead to death if the vomiting is not stopped.

Symptom Pattern C: In this condition, the patient vomits only clear liquid. The patient's face is very pale and the arms and legs are cold. When breathing out, cold is felt when placing your hand under his or her nose. These symptoms may indicate a dangerous "overcooling" condition.

Symptom Pattern D: Vomiting from motion sickness, such as car or sea-sickness.

Treatment

• *Treatment for Vomiting, Symptom Pattern A*

Step One: Apply needle to PC-6 and ST-36.

Step Two: Apply needle to CV-22.

Step Three: Apply needle to CV-12 and then apply indirect moxa to CV-12. If the patient does not recover after this step, apply 7 direct moxa 1/2 rice grain size) to *Jung Kuie*.

• *Treatment of Vomiting, Symptom Pattern B*

Apply 5 direct moxa (red bean size) to PC-5. If the vomiting does not stop, apply 3 direct moxa (red bean size) to PC-7 and 10 direct moxa (red bean size) to ST-18. This treatment will definitely bring about recovery.

• *Treatment of Vomiting, Symptom Pattern C*

Step One: Apply 10 direct moxa (red bean size) to PC-5.

Step Two: Apply 7 direct moxa (red bean size) to CV-12.

Step Three: Apply 3 direct moxa (red bean size) to CV-6, and 5 direct moxa to CV-17.

Note: If after any of the above treatments the patient has not recovered, apply 7 direct moxa (red bean size) to BL-21, and then apply 5 direct moxa (red bean size) to SP-6 and PC-6.

• *Treatment of Vomiting, Symptom Pattern D*

Apply 3-5 direct moxa (green bean size) to GV-20 and PC-5 twice a week for two weeks.

Assistant Points: SP-1, SP-4, PC-3, CV-13, CV-11, BL-17, CV-16, CV-12, GV-14.

Prognosis: Any of the conditions of vomiting (A, B, C or D) requires 1 to 3 treatments.

Vomiting Blood — Hematemesis

Causes: Cancer or ulcer in the stomach; inflammation of the stomach; the menses is vomited through the mouth; illness of the liver or spleen; a blow to the stomach; emotional or psychic stress.

Symptoms: Blood is vomited from the stomach. If much blood is vomited, it will cause the patient to become very anemic, and the condition may become serious.

Special Diagnosis: It is important to distinguish between vomiting blood from the stomach and spitting blood from the lungs. These may be determined according to the following symptomology:

When blood is vomited from the stomach, the patient will describe his or her illness as emanating from the stomach. He or she will have been dizzy before vomiting; the blood will be vomited in one lump, and will be mixed with food and sour smelling; after vomiting blood, the patient's feces has a dark color and seems oily, due to blood in the intestines mixing with the feces.

When blood is expectorated from the lungs, the patient will usually have had a cough for some time before blood had begun to appear in the sputum, and will report having had some illness in the lungs or in the heart; the blood will come out with coughing, and itchiness in the throat. The blood in these cases is always foamy (with tiny bubbles), shows a fresh red color, is mixed with some phlegm, and has a salty odor.

Treatment

Step One: Apply needle to PC-6 and LU-5.

Step Two: Apply needle to ST-36a and SP-1. Use either a thick needle or triangular needle to obtain a strong stimulus from SP-1 (*without* drawing blood), or apply 1 or 2 direct moxa 1/2 rice grain size) to SP-1.

Step Three: Apply needle to BL-20, BL-21, and BL-18. Obtain only a gentle stimulus from BL-18, moving the needle slowly and gently up and down in this point for 30 seconds.

Step Four: Apply needle to CV-13, CV-10, and CV-12; use gentle stimulus on CV-12 for 10 to 20 seconds.

Step Five: Apply indirect moxa with ginger to CV-13, CV-12, and CV-10.

Prognosis: One treatment will stop the vomiting of blood, and 3 treatments will cure the condition. If the patient has not completely recovered after the third treatment, continue with 3 more treatments. If after this time the patient is still vomiting blood, it will be necessary to reexamine the patient to ascertain the origin of the bleeding. The patient may, for example, be suffering from cancer of the stomach or stomach ulcers, in which case the treatment will be specific to the cause.

Visceroptosis — Gastroptosis

Causes: This illness is divided into *prenatal* and *postnatal.* The *prenatal* patient has been very weak from infancy through adulthood. The chest is narrow and long, and the visceroptosis develops easily. The *postnatal* patient is a woman who, as a consequence of bearing several children, has developed stretched and flabby abdominal muscles that no longer give sufficient support to the viscera, and that slip down and cause visceroptosis. Tight binding of the abdomen with belts or laces may also force the viscera downwards and cause visceroptosis. Inflammation of any organ in the abdomen may result in this condition.

Symptoms: Normally, the stomach lies just above the umbilicus when it is empty. When it is full of food, the stomach enlarges so that its lower portion reaches below the umbilicus. In cases of visceroptosis, however, the stomach extends below the umbilicus even when it is empty. Other organs in the abdomen will also fall with the stomach. The patient feels heaviness in the upper part of the abdomen and feels that his or her stomach is swollen. There may be palpitations and headaches. Sleep is disturbed, and the appetite poor, accompanied by nausea, vomiting, and tiredness. The doctor notices that the position of the patient's stomach has altered, with the hypogastric region sunken in, and the lower part of the abdomen swollen. Because the intestines usually drop down as a consequence of this condition, the patient suffers from constipation.

Treatment

Step One: Apply needle to PC-6.

Step Two: Apply needle to ST-36.

Step Three: Apply needle to BL-20, BL-21, and BL-22.

Step Four: Apply needle to CV-12, CV-10, CV-11, ST-25, and CV-4, and then continue with indirect moxa or the ''God's Needle'' moxa pole to the points of this step.

Continue with the above treatment daily for about 15 days, with the following additions:

- During the first 3 days, apply 5 direct moxa (red bean size) to CV-12.
- For the next 3 days, apply 5 direct moxa to CV-4.
- For the next 3 days apply 30 moxa to CV-8. If the hole of the umbilicus is deep, fill it with salt and apply moxa on the salt. The moxa upon the salt must be yellow bean size. But if the umbilicus hole is shallow, apply direct moxa (red bean size) to the umbilicus from 10 to 20 times.

If after 9 days the patient has not recovered, apply 5 direct moxa (red bean size) to ST-25 daily for the next 3 days. If the patient still does not recover completely, apply 5 direct moxa (red bean size) to BL-21 for 3 to 5 days. While applying moxa as indicated for the 15 days or more, continue with the 4 steps mentioned earlier for this treatment.

Prognosis: Two to three weeks of daily treatment are required to bring about recovery.

Cancer or Tumor in the Stomach

Symptoms: The symptoms here are very much like those of chronic inflammation of the stomach. The patient has a poor appetite and feels that the upper part of the abdomen is swollen. There is a little pain, and constipation. The whole body is tired; the patient is thin, and vomits regularly at a fixed time in the day or night. By feeling the patient's abdomen, the doctor can distinguish the growth with his or her fingers or hand. The growth will feel round, or elongated and curved, with an irregular surface. If the cancer or growth is at the entrance to the stomach, the patient will find it very difficult to keep food down.

Treatment

Step One: Apply needle to PC-6 and ST-36.

Step Two: Apply needle to CV-12 and CV-10.

Step Three: Apply three needles to the growth, one at each end and a third at the center.

The stimuli obtained in each point of **Step Three** will be strong. After the application of the needles, apply indirect moxa, with ginger or instrument, to the whole region of the growth, until the skin has been heated to a reddish color. It is also effective to burn moxa on the handle of the needles, or to apply electrical stimulation to them for 5 to 10 minutes.

Step Four: Apply 14 direct moxa (red bean size) to XB-1 *(Pee Gun)*. This point is 3 1/2 finger divisions lateral from the point under the twelfth thoracic vertebra.

If the condition is severe, the moxa applied to XB-1 should be yellow bean size. If the growth is on the patient's left side, apply the direct moxa to the left side. If the growth is on the right side, apply direct moxa to the right side. If the growth is on both sides or on the center, apply direct moxa to *(Pee Gun)* on both sides.

Step Five: Apply 10 direct moxa (red bean size) to CV-8. If the hole of the umbilicus is deep, fill it with salt and apply yellow bean size moxa on top of the salt.

If the results of the above steps appear slowly, apply 10 direct moxa (red bean size) to CV-10. The above mentioned steps of treatment must be taken daily, except **Step Four** which must be taken only once in two weeks.

Assistant Points: ST-44 and SP-4.

Prognosis: In the first stages (i.e., non-severe cases), this illness may be cured with 15-30 treatments.

Stomach Ulcer

Causes: Inflammation of a small part of the mucus membrane of the stomach, which has been aggravated by gastric secretions (hydrochloric acid); excessive eating of meat; eating food that is too hot and thereby injures the mucus membrane of the stomach; tuberculosis of the stomach; syphilis. This disease is more common in women than in men, and occurs most often between the ages of 20 and 30.

Symptoms: Cramping pains in the stomach; severe burning or sharp, piercing sensation in the stomach directly below the sternum, always after meals. The location of the ulcer will coincide with the region of pain, which may radiate to the back and feel as though the back is being bitten. When the pain is very severe, the patient vomits. The patient may also vomit after meals. When the ulcer is suppurating, there will be pus or blood mixed with the vomitus. Blood may also come out in the feces and will be black in color. The patient's appetite is good. If constipation exists, it will be slight.

Treatment

Step One: Apply needle to LI-11 and PC-6.

Step Two: Apply needle to SP-10, ST-36, SP-4, and ST-44.

Step Three: Apply needle to BL-21. After the stimulus has been obtained, apply indirect moxa with ginger or instrument.

Step Four: Apply needle to CV-12 and CV-10. Use light stimulus, as the ulcer will be in the vicinity of these points. Then apply indirect moxa to these 2 points until the skin is reddish in color.

Step Five: Apply needle to the most painful place and obtain a mild stimulus. Continue with indirect moxa with the instrument. Do not use the instrument very hot, and apply on the skin very lightly.

The above treatment must be applied daily. In addition, if *and only if* the patient has no fever, apply 5 direct moxa (red bean size) to SP-10 once every five days. If the patient does not recover, alternate between SP-10 and LI-11 every five days. Apply 5 direct moxa on GB-34a. This will be very effective.

Prognosis: In mild conditions approximately 30 treatments are required, and in severe conditions approximately 60 treatments are required.

Cancer or Tumor in the Gallbladder

Symptoms: A growth can be felt in the position of the gallbladder, which is enlarged because of it. The growth extends down towards the umbilicus. There is severe pain in the region of the gallbladder accompanied by mild jaundice. The patient is thin. If the growth enlarges to the extent that it connects itself to the liver, it can be expected that the growth is spreading into that organ.

Treatment

Step One: Apply 10 direct moxa (green bean size) to LV-13, and 5 direct moxa (green bean size) to LV-14, both on the right side of the body.

Step Two: Apply needle to CV-14, CV-12, and BL-19, and then apply indirect moxa to these 3 points.

Step Three: Apply 14 direct moxa (green bean size) to *Pee Gun* on the right side once every seven days.

Step Four: Apply needle to both ends and in the middle of the growth, obtaining a light stimulus in each instance. Then apply indirect moxa with ginger or instrument lightly for about 15 minutes. Do not press the instrument with any force on the region of the gallbladder.

Prognosis: In the first stages of this disease, 10 to 20 treatments are required. If the cancer or growth has enlarged to the extent that it has spread to the liver, it will be very difficult to cure, but it is worth trying. If, in this case, the patient does meet with some degree of success, it should be expected that a cure will take a very long time.

Jaundice — Hepatitis

Causes: Acute inflammation of the stomach or the duodenum; sorrow for a prolonged period; typhoid fever; pneumonia.

Symptoms: The patient's skin, mucus membrane, inside of the mouth, lips, eyeball, and even urine are all a deep yellowish color. The pulse is slow, about 50 beats per minute. The patient suffers from headaches, fatigue, lacks appetite, and suffers from itching of the skin. In some cases there is a little pain in the region of the gallbladder.

Treatment

Step One: Apply needle to PC-6 and SI-4.

Step Two: Apply needle to ST-36.

Step Three: Apply needle to GV-9, BL-18, and BL-19.

Step Four: Apply needle to CV-12, CV-10, KI-16 and LIV-14.

Step Five: After the yellow color has gone, if there is some pain in the right loin, apply 3 direct moxa on LV-13 on the right side of the body.

Note: Do not use moxa in this case.

Prognosis: Three to seven treatments by acupuncture will bring about recovery. To expedite the cure, have the patient take the medicine below.

Prescription for Jaundice		
Herb		Quantity
Chinese	Pharmaceutical Name	
鷄骨草	*Fructus Abri*	2 oz.
紅棗	*Fructus Zizyphi Jujubae*	10 pcs.

Boil the above herbs with 5 bowls of fresh water until reduced to one bowl. Let the patient drink this while the beverage is still warm; this will help the patient very much. In fact, taking this beverage once a day for 10 days will cure the disease.

Cancer or Tumor of the Pancreas

Causes: The cause is not known, but the disease is quite common. The tumor develops at the head of the pancreas, though sometimes it starts in the middle or even the tail of that organ.

Symptoms: Pain in the upper part of the abdomen which is always at a regular time each day. (In these cases, treat according to the Chinese clock). With the growth at the head of the pancreas, it may press against the gallbladder and thereby cause mild jaundice. The growth can be felt on the upper part of the abdomen above the region of the umbilicus. A small pulse may be felt there which corresponds with that of the umbilicus. The patient's feces is without bile and, lacking bile's yellow pigment, is ashen white in color. The patient loses weight rapidly and there may be vomiting.

Treatment

Step One: Apply needle to PC-6 and ST-36.

Step Two: Apply needle to BL-20.

Step Three: Apply needle to CV-12, CV-10, and CV-6.

Step Four: Apply needles at the two ends and in the middle of the growth, obtaining a light stimulus in each place. Continue with indirect moxa with ginger or instrument for 10 to 15 minutes, or burn moxa on the handles of the needles. It is also possible to burn 10 soybean size moxa on CV-10.

Step Five: On the first day of the treatment, and once every seven days thereafter, apply 14 direct moxa (red bean size) to XB-1 *(Pee Gun)*. If the tumor is on the right side of the body, apply on *Pee Gun* of the right side, and vice versa. Use electric stimulation on the growth for 10 minutes and follow with indirect moxa.

Prognosis: In mild conditions or in the first stages, 10 to 20 treatments bring about a cure. Severe cases tend to be incurable.

Neuralgia of the Intestines

Causes: Eating or drinking in excess; too much gas in the intestines; retaining the feces in too great a quantity or for too long; worms in the intestines.

Symptoms: Sudden severe pain in the intestines. The patient prefers to lie on his or her stomach rather than his or her back; cold sweat and vomiting during the period of pain; difficulty in breathing; palpitations; frequent urination. Occasionally there will be cramping in the calf or in the whole body. The pains come on for a few minutes to a few hours and then will stop. After a few days there is a return of the pains. In the intervening period (i.e., between the bouts of pain), the patient feels perfectly normal.

Treatment

Step One: Apply needle to ST-36.

Step Two: Apply needle followed by indirect moxa (either with ginger or instrument) to ST-25, CV-6, and CV-4. If the pain does not stop, apply needle to ST-27 and then use indirect moxa to these points.

Step Three: If the condition is severe and the patient does not recover, apply 3 direct moxa (green bean size) to ST-36, ST-25, and CV-4.

Assistant Points: CV-8, LV-8, CV-12, KI-16, GV-4, SP-6, LV-1.

Prognosis: 1 to 3 treatments.

Inflammation of the Intestines with Diarrhea — Enteritis

Causes: Patients with weak bodies are subject to this illness. It may be caused by germs; very hard feces; swallowing fruit pits or other undigestible objects; worms in the intestines that touch the mucus membranes of the intestines thus causing inflammation; eating stale or decomposed food, or eating foodstuff unsuitable for the intestines; consuming mixed cold and hot foods; overeating.

Symptoms: The patient feels swelling in the lower part of the abdomen, with some pain and diarrhea. If the illness goes to the stomach, the patient will vomit. In mild conditions, the patient moves the bowels 20 to 30 times a day. In most cases the patient does not have a fever, however, some patients will have fever and thirst, as well as coldness in the arms and legs. Inflammation of the intestines always occurs first in the ileum. If the inflammation enters the small intestine, the feces will show undigested food. If there is inflammation of the large intestines, the diarrhea will be mixed with feces. If the inflammation involves the duodenum, the patient will also have jaundice. If the inflammation goes down to the rectum, the anus will feel very heavy.

Treatment

Step One: Apply needle to ST-36.

Step Two: Apply needle to CV-12, ST-25, CV-6, and CV-4, and then continue with indirect moxa to these points.

Step Three: Apply 10 moxa to CV-8. If the umbilicus is deep, fill with salt and apply yellow bean size moxa on the salt. If the umbilicus is shallow, apply 5 direct moxa (red bean size) to the umbilicus.

Step Four: If the patient vomits, apply needle to LI-4 and PC-6.

Step Five: If the patient has a heavy, dragging feeling in the anus, apply needle to GV-1 and the feeling will cease immediately.

Assistant Points: GV-20 (with direct or indirect moxa — only for long-term diarrhea), CV-10, BL-20, BL-54, BL-25, and BL-27 are all quite useful in the treatment of diarrhea.

Prognosis: 1 to 3 treatments will bring about recovery.

Prescription for Enteritis	
Step One	Pound 1 or 2 pieces of fresh ginger.
Step Two	Place pounded ginger just above the eyebrows, over the nose and around the eyes.

This will help to relieve the diarrhea, and is even effective in cases of cholera. This prescription is required only in severe conditions, as the needle and moxa alone will otherwise suffice.

Inflammation of the Caecum — Appendicitis —

Causes: Germs in the caecum; constipation; sedentary occupations.

Symptoms: In the acute condition, there are no warning signs of the illness. The attack is sudden, with severe pain felt first at the base of the abdomen, on the inside corner of the ileum on the right side. The pain radiates upward toward the gallbladder. When the pain is very severe, the patient may vomit or faint. In chronic conditions, before an attack of pain, the patient has a poor appetite, discomfort in the lower part of the abdomen, and constipation. There is pain on the inside corner of the ileum on the patient's right side. Sometimes the pain is recurrent. If the patient moves or coughs the pain is more severe. The patient has a high fever (approximately 38 °C), poor appetite, hiccoughs or vomiting, coating on the tongue, and offensive breath. The patient is tired and weak. Touching the right lower side of the abdomen, the doctor will find the painful spot and feel a lump like a sausage. Some relief is obtained after moving the bowels. If the inflammation becomes more severe and spreads out, the whole region will become inflamed, and the illness will become worse.

Special Diagnosis: When there is pain between the ileum and the caecum, palpation of the region will increase the pain. Upon palpation, the region is found to be swollen like a sausage, and there will be high fever and vomiting. Before the illness comes on, the patient suffers from constipation. When the patient raises or moves his or her right leg, there is pain in the abdomen. If the inflammation has spread throughout the region, the patient will feel cold and will shiver, and hard irregular lumps will be felt in the region of the caecum. If there is pus in the caecum, the patient will feel very cold and will shiver, his or her fever will go up to 40 °C, and severe local pain will be felt. The patient will have the desire to bend the knee by drawing in his or her leg and letting the knee stick out. If there is still some pain in the caecum when the patient moves his or her bowels, with a high temperature and peritonitis one week after the onset of the disease, you will know that there is pus in the caecum.

Treatment

Step One: Apply needle to ST-36, SP-10, and SP-1 (with strong stimulus on SP-1).

Step Two: Apply needle to the right side of the abdomen on ST-25, ST-29, and the spot where the pain is severe (obtain only a light stimulus from the painful spot).

Step Three: Apply needle to BL-54.

If the pain does not cease after step three, continue with the following step:

Step Four: Apply 5 direct moxa 1/2 rice grain size) to LV-1 and XT-1 *(Tu Yin)*.

Assistant Points: XA-2 (*Jhow Jian,* on the point of the elbow), XA-1 (*Erh Bai,* 4 divisions up from PC-7, between two tendons and one at the outer side of the tendons), CV-5 and LI-11. Of these points the most useful are *Erh Bai* (with needle) and *Jhow Jian* (with 7 red bean size direct moxa).

Prognosis: In mild conditions, 5-7 treatments should suffice. Appendicitis with pus in the caecum is very difficult to cure.

Hemorrhage of the Intestine (Blood Comes through the Anus)

Causes: A blow to the abdomen; ulcer in the intestines; internal piles; illness in the heart, liver, or blood vessels; or worms in the intestines.

Symptoms: If much blood is lost, the patient may faint. The face is pale and the patient has a cold sensation in the arms and legs. The pulse is weak. When the blood flows out there will be some slight pain in the intestines. The blood may either appear mixed with the feces (indicating that its origin is the small intestine), or as a fresh, red-like liquid. If the patient suffers from constipation, the blood will be black in color. If the bleeding originates in the ileum, blood will come out after the feces and fall upon it. If blood and feces come out together, and the patient also vomits blood, this indicates hemorrhage of the stomach and not the intestine. If the blood comes out before the feces, there is bleeding in the rectum.

Treatment

Step One: Apply needle to ST-36 and PC-6.

Step Two: Apply needle to ST-25 and CV-4.

Step Three: Apply needle to BL-17 and GV-1.

Step Four: Apply 7 direct moxa (red bean size) to GV-4. If the patient is a young man under 20 years of age, substitute a needle for the moxa on this point to avoid overheating him.

Step Five: Apply 7 direct moxa (red bean size) to the two points one finger division on both sides of GV-4.

Continue with the above treatment daily for a few days, and if the patient does not improve apply 14 direct moxa (green bean size) to GV-1.

Assistant Points: PC-8, SP-4, SP-5.

Prognosis: Three to five treatments should cure the patient.

Tuberculosis in the Intestines

Causes: This condition is always related to tuberculosis of the lungs. Seldom does one find a case of tuberculosis in the intestines which is not related to tuberculosis in the lungs, except in babies and very small children who have taken food from tuberculosis patients.

Symptoms: In its early stages, this illness is very difficult to diagnose. The patient suffers from morning diarrhea and pain in the lower part of the abdomen (where there will be lumps), and will have a high fever. The feces show undigested food and are always mixed with a little blood and pus.

Treatment

Step One: Apply 3 direct moxa (green bean size) to GV-20.

Step Two: Apply needle to ST-36.

Step Three: Apply needle to BL-20.

Step Four: Apply needle to ST-25, CV-6, and CV-4. Continue with indirect moxa with instrument to these points as well as to the lumps on the lower part of the abdomen until the skin changes to a reddish color.

Step Five: Apply 20 moxa (yellow bean size) with salt to CV-8.

Prognosis: In the early stages, it is easy to cure, but the number of treatments required cannot be stated. If the tuberculosis has spread, and there are many lumps in the intestines, the condition will be very difficult to cure.

Dysentery

Causes: There are two types of dysentery, *amoebic* (or *tropical*) and *bacillary*. Both are caused by contaminated food or drink, or by flies introducing the germs into the body.

Symptoms: The feces comes out like jelly with red blood mixed in it, accompanied by pain in the abdomen and inflammation and a heavy feeling in the rectum.

Bacillary dysentery begins like catarrh of the intestines. After 2 to 5 days the patient will find that he or she has dysentery. On other occasions, the dysentery will come on suddenly. Most patients do not have a fever, but a low grade fever may accompany this disease.

Amoebic dysentery always comes on suddenly, with pain in the abdomen and inflammation and heavy feelings in the rectum. Although some patients have a slight fever, most patients will not. Dysentery without fever is more difficult to cure. If the patient is not cured within a few months, dropsy will develop, which may be fatal.

Treatment

Step One: Apply needle to LI-4 and ST-36.

Step Two: Apply needle to BL-20 and GV-1.

Step Three: Apply needle to CV-12, ST-25, CV-4, and CV-6. If the patient has no fever, continue with indirect moxa to the points of **Step Three.**

Prognosis: In adults, neither form of dysentery is extremely dangerous. However, for infants, children, and the elderly, dysentery is a particularly serious illness. Vomiting and hiccoughing during dysentery indicate that the condition is very serious and will be difficult to cure. In mild conditions 2-3 treatments will suffice. In severe conditions, 7 or more treatments will be needed.

Prescription for Amoebic Dysentery	
Step One	Break the shell and extract the seed of *Ya Dan Tzi* (Fructus Brucea). Squeeze the seed between two pieces of paper to extract the oil.
Step Two	Sprinkle with corn starch, and swallow (do not chew) 3 pieces with half a glass of warm water daily.

Prescription for Bacillary Dysentery		
Herb		Quantity
Chinese	Pharmaceutical Name	
枳實	*Fructus Ponciri*	9 grams
甘草	*Radix Glycyrrhiza*	9 grams
柴胡	*Radix Bupleuri*	9 grams
白芍	*Radix Paeonia Lactiflora*	9 grams
薤白	*Bulbus Allii Chinensis*	9 grams
白頭翁	*Radix Pulsatillae*	9 grams

Boil the above herbs in three cups of water under low heat until one cup remains. Drink when warm, once daily for three days.

The traditional Chinese pharmacist uses the *Ch'ien* (錢) (equal to approximately 3 grams) as the basic unit for weighing herbs in prescriptions.

Constipation

Causes — acute and chronic: Acute constipation may be a symptom of another disease, and is generally treated as part of an overall treatment plan. Chronic constipation, however, is a condition in itself, and must be treated directly. Constipation is more common in women than in men. Those who lead a sedentary, irregular, or rushed existence are more prone to constipation.

Symptoms: A healthy person will move their bowels once or twice daily; even once in two days can be considered normal. A bowel movement only once in three days, as well as daily diminishing of the quantity of the feces, are signs of constipation.

In chronic conditions, the patient will have heaviness, swelling, and some discomfort in the abdomen. There will be lack of appetite as well as eructation, a little congestion and dizziness in the head. In severe conditions, the patient will not respond even to a strong purgative. Lumps of feces can be felt by palpation in the abdomen. If the feces remains too long in the abdomen, the patient will develop intestinal ulcers, and may even have peritonitis through the ulcers. If the feces remain in the rectum too long, piles will result.

Treatment

Step One: Apply needle to TW-6.

Step Two: Apply needle to LV-3, LV-1, and BL-57.

Step Three: Apply needle to BL-25 and GV-1.

Step Four: Apply needle to CV-6, CV-4, KI-16, and ST-25.

Step Five: Apply 5 direct moxa (green bean size) to LV-13.

Prognosis: In acute conditions, 1 or 2 treatments will suffice. In chronic conditions, 7 to 10 treatments should suffice.

Piles — Hemorrhoids

Causes: The hemorrhoidal vein lies in the region of the anus. When blood is prevented from moving out of this vein, piles will ensue. Chronic constipation, certain diseases of the uterus, bladder, or ovary, overuse of purgatives, sedentary habits, horseback riding for too long, and excessive smoking or drinking may all contribute to exacerbate hemorrhoidal blood flow.

Symptoms: There are three types of piles: *internal, middle,* and *external.* In *external* piles, the patient will feel some change in the anus, followed by itching, hot sensations and later pain, but no bleeding. Lumps about the size of peanuts are noticeable. With *internal* piles, the patient will not feel any discomfort in the beginning, but gradually will feel some difference inside the anus, followed by itching, hot sensations, pain, and heaviness. Constipation will follow. When the condition becomes severe there will be bleeding. *Middle* piles is really a form of outer piles, except that in this condition the piles are at the anus, or just a little inside. When the anus opens or the feces come out this type of pile shows itself.

Special Diagnosis: If the patient has piles in the anus, there will be a small piece of tissue, like a pimple or wart between the upper gum and the upper lip. One such "pimple" means one pile, more means more piles.

Treatment

Step One: Apply needle to BL-57 and BL-60.

Step Two: Apply needle to XA-1 *(Erh Bai)* and PC-4.

Step Three: Apply 5 direct moxa (red bean size) to PC-4.

Step Four: Apply needle to GV-4 and GV-1. If the patient suffers from outer piles also apply **Step Five**.

Step Five: Apply 5 direct moxa (red bean size) to the pile, but do not burn the moxa all the way down; as soon as the patient feels pain, withdraw the moxa.

Step Six: If the piles are difficult to cure apply 7 direct moxa (green bean size) to GV-1.

Note: Apply the above steps daily, except that 5 direct moxa (red bean size) to PC-4 should be applied only once every 5 days.

Anal Fistula and Rectal Prolapse

Two disorders that result directly from piles, and that require special treatment, are *Anal Fistula,* piles that have decayed over a long period of time and have opened a hole next to the anus, and *Prolapse of the Rectum,* a chronic condition of piles causing prolapse of the anus.

Treatment

• *Treatment of Anal Fistula*

Step One: Mix powdered *Fu Zi* (Radix Aconitum) with enough warm water to make a number of small cakes, each slightly larger than the hole of the fistula.

Step Two: Cover the hole of the fistula with this cake, and apply yellow bean size moxa on the cake until it has dried up.

Step Three: Remove the dried cake and replace with a fresh one. Repeat procedure until 3 cakes have been used.

Perform the above treatment 2 or 3 times each day until the patient's flesh has filled the hole made by the fistula. During the treatment, apply 5 moxa (red bean size) on SP-10 once each day for 5 days.

• *Treatment of Rectal Prolapse*

Step One: Apply 5 direct moxa (red bean size) to GV-20.

Step Two: Apply 7 direct moxa (red bean size) to GV-1.

Step Three: Apply moxa with salt to CV-8. The number of moxa applied should equal the patient's age in years.

After treatment the patient should remain in bed for 7 days and not get up at all. During this time a bed pan should be used. This treatment for prolapse of the rectum should continue daily for three days after which the patient should recover.

Prognosis: In mild conditions, 1 to 3 treatments; the piles should subside in one or two months without further treatment. If the patient has not recovered completely after this period, one or two additional treatments should be given. In chronic or severe conditions, daily treatment for about 10 to 14 days is required.

Diabetes

Causes: Heredity; obesity; chronic constipation; rheumatism; old age. Men are more prone to this ailment than women, and it is more common after middle age.

Symptoms: The patient's blood has too much sugar, as indicated by urinalysis. The patient gets thinner from day to day. The three special symptoms in the diabetic are: *excessive urine, insatiable hunger,* and *insatiable thirst.*

In severe conditions, the patient also suffers from neuritis or neuralgia, inflammation of the retina of the eye which may lead to dimness of vision or partial blindness, and lessened sexual desire or impotence. In mild conditions, blood sugar can be controlled with diet, and specifically by avoiding consumption of sugar and simple carbohydrates. In conditions of medium severity, the patient should also avoid food with albumin. In severe conditions, diabetes cannot be controlled by diet.

Treatment

Step One: Apply needle to KI-2.

Step Two: Apply needle to BL-13, BL-20, BL-21, BL-22, and BL-23. Apply 5 moxa (red bean size) to CV-4.

Step Three: If the patient suffers from intense thirst, in addition to steps one and two, apply needle to HT-7, CV-24, GV-26, XF-7 *(Hai Chuen)* and XF-8 *(Jin Jin, Yu Yeh)*. Draw out a few drops of blood from this last point.

Step Four: For cases in which the patient suffers from intense hunger, in addition to applying **Step One** and **Step Two**, apply needle to LU-9, ST-36, and ST-44. Apply 5 direct moxa (red bean size) on CV-12.

Step Five: When the patient suffers from polyuria, after applying **Step One** and **Step Two**, apply needle to GV-2, and 5 direct moxa on GV-4 and BL-23.

Assistant Points: ST-33, LV-2, LV-1.

Prognosis: About 20 treatments are required to effect a cure.

Prescription I for Diabetes	
Step One	Take a piece of raw ginger the width of two fingers and burn it with charcoal in a charcoal stove until the skin of the ginger is all black.
Step Two	Take the ginger out and allow to cool sightly. The ginger will still be hot.
Step Three	Scrape off the burnt skin of the ginger completely and eat the remaining part of the ginger while it is still hot.

Prescription II for Diabetes	
Step One	Clean a fresh pancreas of a pig and cut into small pieces the size of a yellow bean.
Step Two	Eat six to eight of the tiny pieces of raw pancreas, swallowed with warm water, every day, 3 times daily.
Step Three	Allow the patient to take more of the raw pancreas if he or she can be persuaded to do so, as this will be found a great help toward the cure.

Water in the Abdomen
Dropsy — Acites

Causes: Disease of the heart or lungs; inflammation of the kidneys; cancer; tuberculosis; cirrhosis of the liver; inadequate blood circulation (particularly the portal circulation of the liver).

Symptoms: Dropsy is difficult to diagnose in its early stages. The abdominal and systemic swelling in dropsy is different from the swelling of peritonitis, and the fever of the latter is absent. When the patient lies down, the top center of the abdomen will flatten, and the swelling will show more on the sides of the abdomen. When the patient stands, the lower part of the abdomen swells a great deal. The skin gets thin and shiny, and in the lower part of the abdomen there will be stretch lines similar to those of a woman after pregnancy. The umbilicus will fill up, though with some patients the umbilicus will remain well defined. If the water in the abdomen remains for many days, it will cause the veins to become prominent. The patient's legs and genitals will also swell.

Treatment

• ***The following points require daily treatment***:

Step One: Apply needle to GV-26.

Step Two: Apply needle to BL-23 and continue with indirect moxa. If the condition is severe, apply 5 direct moxa (red bean size).

Step Three: Apply needle to CV-12, CV-9, CV-7, CV-6, CV-4, ST-28, and continue with indirect moxa to each of these points until the skin is red. If the condition is severe, apply 7 direct moxa (red bean size) to CV-9 and/or CV-4.

• ***In addition to the above treatment, the following two steps are to be used on alternate days:***

Step Four: **First day:** Apply needle to SP-9, SP-6, and ST-36. Apply indirect moxa to all these points. If the condition is severe, apply 5 direct moxa (red bean size) to SP-9.

Step Five: **Second day:** Apply needle to KI-6, KI-7, and KI-8, and then apply indirect moxa to these points until the skin is red. If the condition is severe, apply 5 direct moxa (red bean size) to KI-6.

Step Six: If there is difficulty with urination, apply 20-30 moxa on CV-8.

Note: Patients suffering from dropsy must not eat salty foods, cold foods, vegetables, or fruits, and they must limit their intake of water.

Prognosis: In mild conditions of dropsy, about 10 treatments are required. In severe conditions, 20 to 30 treatments will be necessary.

Prescription for Dropsy	
Step One	Remove the skin from 1 1/4 lbs of dry garlic and boil with two small eels, each the thickness of two fingers, for two hours in a container containing about 4 lbs of water. The amount of liquid will be greatly reduced.
Step Two	Eat some of the eel and garlic, and drink as much of the juice as is reasonable. This will help greatly to cure the dropsy.

Inflammation of the Bladder

Causes: Germs entering the bladder as a result of some infectious diseases; trauma to the abdomen; inflammation of some organ next to the bladder.

Symptoms: This illness is divided into *acute* and *chronic.*

In the *acute* condition, the patient has both fever and feelings of chill; the bladder as well as the region between the scrotum and the anus feels painful; frequent urination is accompanied by dysuria and incomplete voidance. If the condition suddenly becomes severe, there will be pus in the bladder which will be passed during urination.

In the *chronic* condition the patient has no fever. He or she urinates frequently and with discomfort. The urine itself is cloudy. The patient is always miserable and does not like to sit down. The patient becomes thinner, and if this condition lasts for a long time, other dangerous diseases will develop.

Treatment

Step One: Apply needle to SP-9 and SP-6.

Step Two: Apply needle to BL-22, BL-23, BL-27, BL-28, BL-31, BL-32, BL-33, and BL-34.

Step Three: Apply needle to CV-6, CV-4, and ST-28.

In acute conditions, only needle to the above points; in chronic conditions, follow the needle application with indirect moxa.

Prognosis: In acute conditions, 2 or 3 treatments will suffice. In chronic conditions, 7 to 10 treatments are required.

Numbness of the Bladder

Numbness of the bladder involves two distinct symptom patterns: *the inability to urinate (anuria)* and *incontinence*.

Causes: Illness of the spinal cord; infectious disease; inflammation of the urinary bladder; cancer in the bladder; excessive masturbation; excessive sexual intercourse; numbness of the bladder nerves that control urination.

Symptoms accompanying the inability to urinate: If the nerve controlling bladder function is numb, the intervals between urination will become greater. In severe conditions, the patient feels that although the bladder is filled with urine it cannot be passed. Although the patient uses the muscles of the abdomen to press on the bladder, only a few drops may come out, and the bladder will swell up.

Symptoms accompanying incontinence: When the patient coughs or sneezes or laughs, the urine will come out freely.

Treatment

• ***Treatment of inability to urinate due to numbness of the bladder***

Step One: Apply needle to ST-36, SP-9, SP-6, and LV-8.

Step Two: Apply needle to CV-6, CV-4, CV-3, CV-2, and ST-28. If the patient is ''overheated'' the above treatment will suffice, but if the patient if ''overcooled,'' in addition to the above apply 5 direct moxa (green bean size) to SP-6 and 10 moxa to CV-8.

• ***Treatment of incontinence due to numbness of the bladder***

Step One: Apply needle to SP-9 and SP-6.

Step Two: Apply needle to CV-6 and CV-4.

Step Three: Apply needle to BL-22 and BL-23.

Step Four: After the above treatment, continue with 5 direct moxa (red bean size) to BL-23 and CV-4.

Note: This illness is always an "overcooling" condition.

Assistant Points: BL-31, BL-32, BL-33, BL-34, CV-7, CV-2, GV-1, BL-30, LU-5, HT-7, KI-1, ST-40, BL-54, LV-3.

Prognosis: In mild conditions, 2 or 3 treatments. In severe conditions, 7 to 10 treatments are necessary.

Stones in the Urinary Bladder or Kidney

Causes: Small stones from the kidney enter the urinary bladder, and the chemical composition in the urine combines with the small stones so that they grow larger and larger in size; eggs of worms or seeds of fruit enter the bladder, mix with chemicals in the bladder and develop into small stones. Sometimes there is only one stone in the bladder; sometimes there are many; some stones are like grains of sand while others become as large as an egg. Patients who have stones in the bladder also develop stones in the kidney.

Symptoms: The symptoms will depend on the size of the stone. The first signs are pain in the region between the anus and the scrotum, with a constant desire to urinate. The urine is sometimes colored with a little blood. If the patient gets up and walks or uses strength to do something, the pain will increase, and it will go up to the tip of the penis, anus, and thighs. When the patient lies down and draws up his or her legs the pain will decrease. When the patient passes urine the flow may suddenly stop and the stoppage is followed with pain, because the stone has blocked the hole of the bladder. If the patient bends on one side of his body the pain will cease as soon as the stone no longer blocks the hole. If the stone is in the kidney, the patient will feel severe low back pain.

Treatment

- ***Treatment of kidney and urinary bladder stones***

Step One: Apply needle to SP-9 and SP-6.

Step Two: Apply needle to KI-6, LV-1, and KI-1.

Step Three: Apply 10 red bean size moxa directly or upon salt to CV-8.

Step Four: Apply 3 direct moxa (red bean size) to SP-6 and LV-2, one point for each day, and 14 direct moxa (green bean size) on XB-1 *(Pee Gun).*

Step Five: Apply 10 direct moxa (green bean size) to BL-23 and GV-4.

- *Treatment of Gallbladder Stone*

Step One: Apply needle to BL-18 and BL-19.

Step Two: Apply 14 direct moxa (yellow bean size) on right side of XB-1 *(Pee Gun)*.

This treatment should be given once a week, and continued for 4 to 6 weeks.

Prognosis: In mild conditions, when the stones are the size of grains of sand, 5 to 10 treatments are necessary; in chronic conditions about 30 to 40 treatments are necessary. If each stone is as large as an egg, it is very difficult to cure through acupuncture.

Prescription for Stones	
Step One	Boil 5 lbs. of *Che Chen Tsao* (Herba Plantaginis) in 7 lbs. of water down to 1 lb. of liquid.
Step Two	Drink the entire dose, and repeat for several days.

Bedwetting

Causes: This illness occurs commonly in children between the ages of 3 and 12, and may be due to malnutrition, general debility, emotional upset, intestinal parasites, or withering of the kidneys.

Symptoms: The child urinates when sleeping. After going to bed and falling asleep, the child dreams of passing urine, and actually does so in bed. This illness is rare in adults.

Treatment

Step One: Apply needle to SP-9 and SP-6.

Step Two: Apply needle to BL-23, GV-4, GV-2. In mild conditions apply indirect moxa with ginger to BL-23. In severe conditions apply 5 direct moxa (green bean size) to BL-23.

Step Three: Apply needle to CV-4, and continue with indirect moxa with ginger to that point. In severe cases, apply 5 direct moxa (green bean size) to CV-4.

Assistant Points: HT-7, HT-5, BL-54, KI-2, LV-1, BL-25, BL-27.

Prognosis: In mild conditions, about 3 treatments; in chronic conditions, 7 to 10 treatments.

Withering of the Kidneys

Causes: Excessive eating and drinking; inflammation of the kidneys; syphilis; gonorrhea; malaria.

Symptoms: In the beginning there are no signs and no pain. In some cases, however, the illness will come on suddenly. In the beginning of the illness the patient has palpitations, headache, dizziness, nose-bleeding, vomiting, dimness of vision, and sometimes fainting. These symptoms may be puzzling, and may at first appear to indicate some other disorder. The first important corroborating sign is frequent and copious passing of urine during the night. If the patient's condition continues to deteriorate, dropsy will also develop, which will start in the face and gradually spread throughout the entire body.

Treatment

Step One: Apply needle to SP-9, SP-6 and KI-2, and apply 7 moxa (green bean size) on KI-2.

Step Two: Apply needle to BL-22 and BL-23, and then apply 7 direct moxa (red bean size) to BL-23.

Step Three: Apply needle to CV-6 and CV-4, and then apply 5 direct moxa (red bean size) to CV-4.

Note: If the patient's condition has developed into dropsy, use only the treatment for dropsy.

Prognosis: If the condition has not developed into dropsy, 5 to 10 treatments will bring about recovery.

Inflammation of the Kidney

Causes: Infectious disease; pregnancy; catching cold.

Symptoms: The principal sign is severe decrease in urine which may reach a stage when there is no urine for several days. The urine is turbid, and changes into the color of tea mixed with a little blood, the juice of fresh beef, or the color of blood itself, red and dark. In advanced stages, this condition may be accompanied by dropsy, beginning in the eyelids and with swelling of the face, and eventually affecting the entire body. The patient has no fever as a rule, though with some there is a mild fever with cold feeling. There is pain in the back in the region of the kidneys. The patient desires to urinate day and night. In some patients, the ability to urinate is unaffected, though when they do, the urine is colored with blood. Other patients will be unable to pass urine at all. If the condition becomes severe, the patient will be subject to vomiting, diarrhea, poor appetite, headache, drowsiness, and may suffer from cramp in the arms and legs. As the condition becomes chronic, it becomes less dangerous, and there will not be as many serious symptoms.

Treatment

Step One: Apply needle to GV-26.

Step Two: Apply needle to KI-2, KI-6, KI-7, and SP-9.

Step Three: Apply needle to GV-4, BL-23, and BL-28.

Step Four: Apply needle to CV-6 and CV-4.

Prognosis: In mild conditions, 5 to 7 treatments and patient will recover. In severe and chronic conditions, 10 to 20 treatments are required.

Inflammation of the Spinal Cord

Causes: Physical strain; sleeping on a cold spot or on the cold ground; injury to the vertebrae; inflammation in the region of the vertebrae; amenorrhea; excessive sexual intercourse; syphilis; infectious disease; lead poisoning.

Symptoms: In the acute condition there is severe pain in the lumbar region and cramp in the nerves of the vertebrae causing an inability to bend the back, a high fever, and paralysis of the legs. In chronic cases, there is a feeling of movement at the tips of the toes. Gradually the patient's legs become paralyzed; paralysis in the rectum and the bladder develops, and the patient is altogether unable to control the passage of urine and feces. If the inflammation of the spinal cord occurs in the thoracic region, there will be paralysis of the upper limbs. If the inflammation occurs in the lumbar region, the paralysis will be in the lower limbs. If the inflammation is in the cervical region of the spinal cord, the whole body will be paralyzed.

Treatment

• ***Treatment of lumbar inflammation and paralysis of the legs***

Step One: Apply needle to BL-23, BL-31, BL-32, BL-33, BL-34 and GV-2.

Step Two: Apply needle to GB-30, GB-31, ST-33, and BL-54.

Step Three: Apply needle to GB-34, ST-36, SP-6, GB-39, KI-3, and BL-60.

Step Four: If the condition is chronic, apply 7 direct moxa (red bean size) to BL-23, BL-31, BL-32, BL-33, BL-34, GB-30, GB-31, GB-34, GB-39, and BL-60 daily for 3 days. The moxa should be applied to two of these points during each treatment until all of the points have been used. Then start back at the beginning again with the first pair.

• ***Treatment of thoracic inflammation and paralysis of the arms***

Step One: Apply needle to GV-14, LI-15, and LI-11.

Step Two: Apply needle to LU-5 and PC-3.

Step Three: Apply needle to LI-10, TW-5, and LI-4.

If the condition is chronic, follow with 5 direct moxa (red bean size) to GV-14, LI-15, LI-11, LI-10, TW-5, and LI-4, each for three consecutive days starting with GV-14.

• ***Treatment of cervical inflammation with general paralysis***

Step One: Follow **Steps One, Two, and Three** for *thoracic inflammation*, above.

Step Two: Apply needle to the points one eye division lateral from between the 3rd and 4th, 4th and 5th, and 5th and 6th cervical vertebrae on both sides of the spine. If the condition is chronic, after applying the needle as indicated above, apply 5 direct moxa (red bean size) to these same points. For the first three days, treat the first of the three points daily; during the next three days, treat the second point; for the next three days, treat the third point. Then repeat the procedure.

Prognosis: In acute conditions, 7 to 10 treatments are necessary. In chronic conditions, 1 to 2 months of daily treatment may be necessary for some recovery. Sometimes this case is very difficult to help, for example if it is the result of a trauma such as a car accident.

Loss of Semen

During sexual intercourse, if the semen comes out too quickly, or if the semen flows out of itself (indicating a more severe condition), loss of semen is indicated.

Causes: Frequent masturbation; excessive sexual intercourse; gonorrhea; excessive amount of foreskin over the tip of the penis; piles; tuberculosis in the lungs; weakness of the nerves of the whole body.

Symptoms: In mild conditions, the semen will be lost once or twice a month. When the penis erects, or when the patient dreams of having sexual intercourse, the semen will flow. In severe conditions, this occurs every night or every other night. Even when the penis merely touches clothes, the semen will come out very easily. In both mild and severe conditions, after the semen flows out the patient will feel very tired and will have headaches, dizziness, palpitations, and feel a lack of efficiency, lack of memory, and lack of appetite. An otherwise healthy young man will not be affected by such loss of semen.

Treatment

Step One: Apply needle to SP-9 and SP-6.

Step Two: Apply needle to BL-15, BL-23, GV-4, and BL-47 and continue with 5 direct moxa (green bean size) to BL-23 and BL-47, one each day.

Step Three: Apply needle to CV-6, CV-4, and CV-3 and continue with 10 direct moxa (green bean size) to CV-3 and/or GV-3.

Step Four: Apply needle to GV-1.

Continue with the above treatment daily for 2 weeks. If the patient does not recover completely, treatment may be continued for up to one more week. If the patient then recovers completely, apply 7 direct moxa (red bean size) to BL-38 and 3 moxa (red bean size) to ST-36. The moxa treatment should continue daily for 3 days and the illness will then not return. Be sure not to apply direct moxa to CV-4; doing so will make the condition much worse.

Prognosis: In mild conditions, about 10 treatments. In severe conditions, about 30 daily treatments will be necessary.

Withering of the Penis — Impotency —

Causes: In youth, the penis had not grown to its full size; carbuncle on the penis; illness in the testicles; lack of sexual desire in elderly men; marrying too early so that when the man reaches middle age the penis withers; illness in the brain or spinal cord; too frequent sexual intercourse; excessive masturbation; withering of the kidneys; weakness of the nerves of the whole body.

Symptoms: The penis does not erect completely. With some patients, before the penis enters the vagina the semen flows out and the penis becomes smaller. In other conditions, even before the semen flows out into the woman's vagina, the patient's penis becomes soft and small. In severe conditions, the penis cannot erect at all and the patient no longer has a desire for sexual intercourse. In such cases some nervous condition will follow.

Treatment

Step One: Apply needle to SP-9, SP-6, and KI-2.

Step Two: Apply needle to GV-4 and BL-23, and then apply 10 direct moxa (red bean size) to GV-4, 5 direct moxa (red bean size) to BL-23, and 7 direct moxa (red bean size) to KI-2. Divide the moxa treatment in 3 days.

Step Three: Apply needle to CV-6, CV-4, CV-3, and ST-29, and continue with 5 direct moxa (red bean size) to CV-4 and use electric stimulation on these points.

Step Four: Apply 5 direct moxa (1/2 rice grain size) to *Nang Di* (this point is directly under the bottom of the scrotum). If the patient recovers, apply 7 direct moxa (red bean size) to BL-38 and 3 direct moxa (green bean size) to ST-36.

Caution: During treatment, and for 100 days thereafter, the patient must not have sexual intercourse and must not arouse sexual desire, so that the penis will be able to regain its strength. If the patient has sexual intercourse during treatment or within 100 days after treatment he will revert to his former condition and a cure will be difficult.

Cramp of the Penis (Penis Retracting into the Abdomen)

Causes: Excessive masturbation before marriage. After marriage, excessive sexual intercourse.

Symptoms: There is suddenly a cramp in the penis and it retracts into the abdomen. The patient is greatly frightened, and his face pale. The patient tries to draw out the penis but is unable to do so.

Treatment

• ***In acute conditions, directly after the onset of the cramp***

Step One: Apply needle to KI-1, BL-57, GV-1, and LV-1. Obtain strong stimulus from GV-1 and retain the needle in that point, moving it lightly in and out for 20 seconds, obtaining the stimulus again and again during this time.

Step Two: Apply needle to CV-6 and CV-4.

Step Three: Apply needle to CV-1.

After these 3 steps, the penis will loosen and come out.

• ***In chronic conditions, when the cramp of the penis has already occurred a number of times during the month, or several times in a week.*** This treatment can be used at the time of the cramp, just after it has occurred, or to prevent its recurrence.

Step One: Apply needle to SP-9, SP-6, and BL-57.

Step Two: Apply needle to CV-6 and CV-4.

Step Three: Apply needle to GV-1 and CV-1.

Step Four: Apply 10 direct moxa (red bean size) to CV-8. If the umbilicus is deep, it should be filled with salt before the moxa is burned, and the moxa should be yellow bean size.

Continue with the above treatment daily for 3 days. From the 4th to the 6th day, apply the needle daily to all of the above points but do not apply more moxa to CV-8. Instead, apply 5 direct moxa (green bean size) to CV-4. From the 7th to the 9th day apply the needle daily to all the points, but no more moxa to CV-8 or CV-4. Instead, apply 5 direct moxa (green bean size) to GV-1. From the 10th to the 12th day apply the needle to all the points but no more moxa to CV-8, CV-4, or GV-1. Apply 7 direct moxa (green bean size) to CV-1. The illness will not return again. During the treatment, and for a month thereafter, the patient must not indulge in sexual intercourse.

Prognosis: Acute conditions, 1 or 2 treatments. Chronic conditions require about 2 weeks of daily treatment.

Inflammation of the Testicles

Causes: Traumatic injury to one or both testicles; gonorrhea; mumps; typhoid fever; rheumatism in the joints.

Symptoms: This ailment is mostly caused by gonorrhea, and appears two to four weeks after the onset of the disease. In this case, usually only one testicle is inflamed. The patient has a fever with feelings of chill, and there will be severe pain in the inflamed testicle. The pain will radiate from the testicle to the base of the penis, up to the lower part of the abdomen or to the region of the sacrum, and/or the upper part of the thighs. The testicle may swell to the size of an egg, or the size of a human fist.

Treatment

• *In acute conditions:*

Step One: Apply needle to SP-10, BL-54, and SP-6.

Step Two: Apply needle to GV-4.

Step Three: Apply needle to LV-1 and then continue with 3 direct moxa (sesame seed or 1/2 rice grain size) to LV-1. If the inflammation of the testicle is on the left, apply direct moxa to LV-1 of the right foot, and vice versa.

Step Four: Apply needle to ST-27 and ST-29 on the same side of the body as the side of the inflamed testicle, and obtain a stimulus to the testicle or scrotum.

Step Five: Apply indirect moxa with ginger to the region that is swollen and painful, that is, next to ST-30.

• *In chronic conditions:*

Step One: Apply needle to SP-9, SP-6, LV-2, and KI-6.

Step Two: Apply needle to LV-1 and continue with 3 direct moxa (1/2 rice grain size). If inflammation is on the left, apply to LV-1 of the right foot, and vice versa.

Step Three: Apply 7 direct moxa (1/2 rice grain size) to XSC-1 *(Nang Di)*. As soon as the flame touches the skin and the patient feels the pain flick off the moxa.

Step Four: If after 5 daily treatments there is no result, apply 7 direct moxa (red bean size) to ST-27 daily for 5 days. Simultaneously continue with the above needle treatment daily, but omit the moxa treatment mentioned earlier. After this, discontinue the direct moxa to ST-27, but continue with 7 direct moxa (red bean size) to ST-29. Continue applying the needle to all points mentioned above. Apply direct moxa to the ST-27 and ST-29 only on the side of the body corresponding to the inflamed testicle.

• *Alternative treatment for chronic conditions:*

Should the above treatment for chronic conditions prove ineffective, apply 5 direct moxa (red bean size) to the point one finger division under BL-57. If the condition is very severe, the moxa should be yellow bean size. This treatment should be given daily for 3 days. After 1 to 2 weeks the disease will gradually disappear.

Prognosis: In acute conditions, 1 to 3 treatments. In chronic conditions, 10 to 20 treatments. If both treatments for chronic conditions are combined the results will be quicker and more satisfactory.

Special Note: After chronic inflammation of one or both testicles, if the swelling has developed to the size of a duck's egg and feels hard like stone, with no pain, and the patient cannot erect the penis, no cure will be possible. This condition is called ''wooden testicle'' by the Chinese.

Dropsy in the Scrotum — Hydrocele —

Causes: Acute condition from a blow to the scrotum; inflammation of the testicles after contracting gonorrhea. The chronic condition develops from the acute condition.

Symptoms: In the acute condition, the scrotum is inflamed and painful, and there may be fever. In the chronic condition, the scrotum is swollen and filled with liquid, but there is neither pain, inflammation, nor fever.

Treatment

Step One: Apply needle to SP-9 and LV-8.

Step Two: Apply needle to LV-3, SP-5, and LV-1.

Step Three: Apply 3 direct moxa (1/2 rice grain size) to LV-1 and 5 direct moxa (green bean size) to SP-5.

Step Four: Apply needle to BL-23 and GV-4. After needle apply 5 direct moxa (green bean size).

Step Five: Apply needle to CV-7, ST-28, and ST-29.

Prognosis: In acute conditions, 3 to 5 treatments. In chronic conditions, 10 to 20 treatments. Chronic cases of hydrocele may be very difficult to treat with acupuncture.

Gonorrhea

Causes: Gonorrhea is contracted in the penis through sexual intercourse with a woman who has the disease, or when the penis comes in contact with clothing or towels used by one who has the disease. Symptoms appear in 1 to 3 days after contact.

Symptoms: The illness is divided into acute and chronic conditions. In the beginning of the acute condition a thick, glue-like liquid passes out from the urethra, and will sometimes block the hole of the penis. There will be difficulty passing urine, with itching, pain, or burning during voidance, as well as frequent desire to urinate. When the condition becomes more severe, the urine will change and become pus-like, and the liquid will be filled with gonorrheal germs. If the disease is not cured, it will soon become chronic. In the chronic condition there will be no pain, but the discharge will continue for as much as ten years or more. After contracting gonorrhea, the patient invariably suffers from inflammation of the bladder and of the testicles, these symptoms frequently continuing even after the patient has been cured.

Treatment

Step One: Apply needle to SP-6 and SP-9. In acute conditions, also apply needle to SP-10 (this point is unnecessary in chronic conditions).

Step Two: Apply needle to BL-23, GV-4, and BL-47. In chronic conditions, apply 5 direct moxa (red bean size) to BL-23; do not apply moxa here for acute conditions.

Step Three: Apply needle to CV-6, CV-4, and CV-3. In chronic conditions, apply 5 direct moxa (red bean size) to CV-3. In acute conditions, apply indirect moxa either with ginger or by instrument to CV-4 and CV-3.

Prognosis: In acute conditions, 3 to 5 treatments will suffice. In chronic conditions, 10 to 15 treatments.

Lymphogranuloma Inguinalis — Bubo —

Causes: This diseases is contracted through sexual intercourse with one who is infected, in the same way as gonorrhea and syphilis.

Symptoms: The inflamed groin is extremely painful, and the patient has a high fever with a cold feeling in the body, lack of appetite, and tiredness throughout the whole body. The sore will enlarge with pus and eventually burst. Sometimes there will be no pus.

Treatment

Step One: Apply needle to SP-6, KI-7, and SP-10.

Step Two Apply needle to BL-54 and BL-57. Obtain a strong stimulus from BL-57 and move the needle in and out for about 10 seconds.

Step Three: Apply indirect moxa with ginger to the inflamed region of the bubo. If the bubo has developed into an ulcer, omit the indirect moxa. Instead, apply 5 direct moxa (red bean size) to SP-10, and apply either the **White Ointment** or **Red Jade Ointment** to the ulcer.

Prognosis: In the first stage, about 3 to 5 treatments will bring about a cure, but if the ulcer has opened up, about 10 treatments will be necessary.

Hernia

Small Intestine Falls Through The Scrotum

A hernia indicates that certain internal organs have moved through a weakness in the muscle wall. Hernia can occur in numerous body sites. This treatment is relevant only for hernias that involve the small intestines dropping down into the scrotum.

Causes: This condition has two origins, *prenatal* and *postnatal*. The *prenatal* condition occurs from incomplete development in utero. The *postnatal* condition is cause by weakening of the abdominal wall, or excessive internal pressure. The usual cause of hernias is excessive strenuous lifting and carrying heavy objects, excessive coughing, or straining at stool. In women it can occur after childbirth, when the abdominal wall is weakened. In the latter case, the hernia will form near the upper thigh or on the white line of the stomach.

Symptoms: In the beginning, there will be a round, sausage-shaped swelling on the abdomen near the upper thigh. Upon lifting or coughing, the hernia may enlarge. You can feel the hernia jump up by pressing the enlarged area and having the patient cough. If the small intestine drops down to the scrotum and the patient stands up, the scrotum will then enlarge. If the patient presses the scrotum while lying down, the small intestine will retract into the abdomen. Even if you don't press on the scrotum, the intestine will retract after fifteen minutes of lying down, accompanied by a sound similar to ''glu-glu, glu-glu.'' When the patient stands, the scrotum will again enlarge. In the first stage of hernia, there will be localized pain. Severe pain accompanies initial movement of the small intestine into the scrotum. After a period of time, however, the patient won't feel pain from this event.

Diagnosis: Hernia must be distinguished from *hydrocele, gas in the scrotum,* and *inflammation of the testicles*.

Inflammation of the testicles is accompanied by local swelling and pain. *Hydrocele* is detected by lifting the scrotum, which is very heavy. When lying down, the scrotum will not become smaller. If you press the scrotum, the water won't retract into the abdomen, and there is no ''glu-glu, glu-glu'' sound. In some of these cases, pressure will not change the size of the scrotum at all. The medical doctor should drain the scrotum to alleviate this condition.

Gas in the scrotum also causes swelling, but does not make the scrotum feel heavy. When the patient lies down its size is not reduced. Pressure on the scrotum should stimulate gas release through the urethra accompanied by the sounds "sze-sze-sze." If there is too much gas in the scrotum, there will be a little pain, but it will not be severe.

Treatment

- ***Treatment of Hernia in the early stages when accompanied by pain***

Step One: Apply 3 moxa to GV-20 (green bean size). Also apply 3 moxa to LV-1 (1/3 long grain rice size). If the condition is on the right side, apply moxa to the left toe; if on the left side, apply moxa on the right.

Step Two: Apply 7 moxa (red bean size) to the point three divisions lateral to CV-4 on the same side as the hernia. This should relieve the pain and help the condition.

- ***Treatment of hernia in advanced conditions without pain***

Step One: Apply needle to LV-8 and ST-30.

Step Two: Apply 5 moxa (1/4 rice grain size) to LV-1 and 5 moxa to *Tu Yin* (on the underside of the second toe in the center of the second crease on both feet).

Step Three: Apply 7 moxa on ST-27 (red bean size). If the hernia is on the right side, apply moxa on the left side and vice versa.

Step Four: Apply 3-5 moxa on GV-20.

Note: The second, third, and fourth steps should be done on three separate days.

Assistant Points: CV-6, CV-4, GB-26 (on the hernia side of the body). You can also treat the special point 4 divisions lateral to CV-5 on the side with the hernia.

Prognosis: In the beginning, this case is easily treated. When the intestine has descended into the scrotum, surgery is advisable.

Agalactia

(Lack of Mother's Milk after Childbirth)

Causes: The mother's body is too weak; the breasts insufficiently developed; the mother is not receiving or absorbing sufficient nourishment.

Symptoms: After childbirth, there is insufficient supply of milk from the breasts.

Treatment

Step One: Apply needle to LI-4, PC-6, and SI-1.

Step Two: Apply needle to SP-6.

Step Three: Apply needle to ST-18 and ST-16. Apply 7 direct moxa (red bean size) to CV-17.

Prognosis: In mild conditions, after 2 or 3 treatments the mother's breasts will be filled with milk. In severe conditions, when the mother has only a few drops of milk from her breasts, 7 to 10 treatments will be necessary. The results in more severe conditions will not be as satisfactory as in mild conditions.

Morning Sickness

(Excessive Vomiting During Pregnancy)

Causes: Internal organs upset by pregnancy.

Symptoms: After being pregnant for 2 to 3 months, a woman may begin to experience nausea and vomiting, which in some cases lasts throughout the entire day. During these bouts, the appetite is suppressed; liquids are often vomited immediately after drinking, though sometimes the patient is able to take in small quantities of solid food. If the vomiting continues for long, the patient will become tired, and will suffer from headaches and insomnia. If the vomiting is severe and persistent, the woman may even die.

Treatment

Step One: Apple needle to PC-6 and PC-5.

Step Two: Apply needle to ST-36, and apply 7 direct moxa (1/2 rice grain size) to XT-1 *(Tu Yin).*

Step Three: Apply needle to CV-22 and CV-12.

Step Four Apply 7 direct moxa (half rice grain size) to XF-2 *(Jung Kuei).*

Step Five: Apply 7 direct moxa (green size) to PC-5.

Prognosis: If the patient's pulse rate ranges from 110 °F to 120 °F, or if the temperature rises to 40 ° C, the patient will be in a serious condition that will be difficult to cure. If the pulse is not fast and the temperature not as high, three to five treatments will bring about recovery.

Irregular Menstruation

Causes: Swelling of the uterus; excessively narrow uterine opening; inflammation of the uterus; inflammation of the ovaries; excessive fatigue; general weakness; neurasthenia.

Symptoms: Uterine or fallopian tube contraction causes intermittent or continuous pain in the lower part of the abdomen, which radiates from the sacrum down to the legs and to the abdomen. If the pain is continuous, inflammation of the uterus or adjacent organs should be suspected. The pain appears either with the onset of the menses, a day or two before the appearance of the menses, or two or three days after onset. Often, when the menses comes, the pain goes away. In other cases, the pain remains until the period of menstruation is over.

Treatment

Step One: Apply needle to SP-6, SP-9, ST-36, and ST-44.

Step Two: Apply needle to BL-23. If there is pain in the sacrum, apply needle to BL-31, BL-32, BL-33, and BL-34, and continue with indirect moxa to these points.

Step Three: Apply needle to ST-25, CV-6, CV-4, and CV-3. Continue with indirect moxa to these points. If the pain is very severe, apply 7 direct moxa (1/2 rice grain size) to XT-1 *(Tu Yin)*. If the pain is below the umbilicus on both sides of the abdomen, apply needle to ST-28 and GB-26, and then continue with indirect moxa.

Prognosis: When the pain is approaching, apply treatment immediately and the pain will cease. It is advisable, however, to continue with daily treatment for 3 or 4 days. After two weeks give one more treatment, followed by a final three day treatment at the time of the next menstrual period. The patient will not be troubled with this illness again.

Absence of Menstruation Through Abnormal Causes

Menstruation begins at approximately 13 years of age, and continues up to the age of 40 or 50. Absence of menses through pregnancy or lactation during this period is natural, and should not be considered a problem. Thus, it is important to be able to recognize the following signs, other than the sudden absence of menstruation, which accompanies pregnancy.

Special Diagnosis — Signs of Pregnancy:

- The skin of the face loses some of its beauty.
- The skin of the body loosens up.
- The respiratory rate is faster than normal.
- Desire for sour foods.
- Casual vomiting after eating.
- The breasts suddenly develop in size.
- The aureole of the breasts darken.
- The passage in the vagina darkens to a slightly purplish color.
- There will be a milky vaginal discharge.
- The passage of the vagina may be slightly swollen.
- The enlarged uterus is pressing against the bladder causes frequent urination, especially at night.

Causes: The organs of reproduction have not developed completely; illness of the ovaries; withering of the mucus membrane inside the uterus; malnourishment; anemia; an infectious illness; severe tuberculosis; chronic inflammation of the kidneys; diabetes; sudden fright; great grief; false pregnancy.

Symptoms: Absence of menses may or may not be accompanied by other signs of illness.

Treatment

Step One: Apply needle to LI-4, SP-6, ST-44, and SP-10.

Step Two: Apply needle to BL-23 and continue with indirect moxa. If the condition is chronic, apply 5 direct moxa (red bean size).

Step Three: Apply needle to ST-25, CV-7, CV-6, CV-4, and CV-3.

Step Four: Apply needle to ST-28 and ST-29.

Step Five: Apply indirect moxa to each of the points of **Step Three** and **Step Four**. If the condition is severe or chronic, apply 5 direct moxa (red bean size) to CV-4.

Prognosis: In acute conditions, one or two treatments will suffice. If menstration has been absent for a few months or longer, over 10 treatments may be necessary.

Hemorrhage of the Uterus Excess Menstrual Flow

Causes: Malnourishment; tuberculosis in the lungs; some illness in the heart, liver, stomach, or reproductive organs; sudden fright or intense grief; irritation due to excessive dancing or horseback riding; excessive sexual intercourse; habitual miscarriage.

Symptoms: When the flow is much heavier than normal, or the period of menstruation lengthens unduly, or if there is menstrual bleeding two or three times in a month, anemia or discharge will result. A very heavy flow of blood unrelated to menstruation is an entirely different condition which, if unchecked, may result in the patient's death.

Treatment

Step One: Apply needle to HT-5.

Step Two: Apply needle to SP-10 and SP-1. Use a thicker needle and obtain a strong stimulus from the SP-1, and then apply 3 direct moxa (1/2 rice grain size) to SP-1.

In mild conditions, one treatment as mentioned above will suffice. In severe and chronic conditions, add the following to the treatment above:

Step Three: Apply thick needle followed by 3 direct moxa (1/2 rice grain size) to LV-1. If patient suffers from severe hemorrhage of the uterus and the blood flows like a spring of water, the moxa must be green bean size. This will be very painful, though it should be explained that after this treatment the flow of blood will lessen considerably or cease altogether. This treatment is very powerful.

Step Four: Apply needle to SP-6 and SP-9.

Step Five: Apply needle to BL-23 and continue with indirect moxa.

Step Six: Apply needle to CV-4 and CV-3, and continue with indirect moxa to these points.

All six steps must be used for patients who suffer from chronically excessive menstruation (i.e., monthly heavy flowing for a long time), too frequent menstruation for a few months, too lengthy periods of menstruation, or menstruation which is continuous, flowing for months.

If the condition is severe, on the first day direct moxa will be applied to LV-1 and SP-1. Direct moxa *must not* be applied on these two points on the second day. Instead, apply 5 direct moxa (red bean size) to SP-10 on the second day; on the third day apply 5 direct moxa (red bean size) to BL-23; on the fourth day apply 5 direct moxa (red bean size) to CV-4. During this period, the needle treatment should be applied daily to the points of **Steps One, Four** and **Six**.

Prognosis: In mild conditions, one or two treatments will suffice. In chronic conditions, about five to seven treatments will suffice. In severe hemorrhage of the uterus, one or two treatments will suffice though three treatments are recommended.

Cramping of the Uterus

Causes: Change of the position of the uterus either by itself, or as a result of acute or chronic inflammation of the ovaries and/or of the fallopian tubes; hysteria; excessive dancing or horseback riding; retaining the urine in the bladder too long; chronic constipation; chilling or wetting of the body directly before or after menstruation; too much heavy manual labor; excessive sexual intercourse.

Symptoms: Uterine cramping, preceded by a feeling of heaviness in the lower part of the abdomen, followed by pain in the lower part of the abdomen and the sacrum which gradually develops into cramping, and which may radiate to the legs as far as the knees. The pain is twisting or piercing, and the patient feels as though a ball inside the abdomen is rising in the direction of the heart. The patient desires to bend her body. When the condition becomes severe, the patient has stomach pains and vomits, and has cramping in the arms, legs, and tongue as well as unconsciousness. The pulse and temperature remain normal.

Treatment

Step One: Apply needle to SP-9, SP-6, and ST-44.

Step Two: Apply needle to BL-57 and KI-1.

Step Three: Apply 7 direct moxa (red bean size) to KI-1. During this procedure, flick off the moxa as soon as the patient feels intense pain. If the condition is very severe, the direct moxa must be completely burnt on this point, and must not be flicked off. Finally, apply 7 direct moxa (1/2 rice grain size) to XT-1 *(Tu Yin).*

Step Four: Apply needle to BL-31, BL-32, BL-33, and BL-34, and continue with indirect moxa to these points.

Step Five: Apply needle to CV-4 and CV-3, and continue with indirect moxa to these points.

Prognosis: In either mild or severe conditions, one or two treatments.

Leukorrhea

Causes: Gonorrhea; vaginal discharge after childbirth associated with anemia; excessive masturbation or sexual intercourse; too much hard physical work that has weakened the body; cold with fever.

Symptoms: In mild conditions, there is only a little yellow or white discharge from the vagina, but there is no sign of illness in other parts of the body. In severe conditions, the mucus membrane of the vagina may be swollen and reddish, with a pressing feeling in the vagina accompanied by some pain, sometimes with vomiting and fever, and frequent passing of urine. It is difficult to have sexual intercourse and to urinate. The liquid discharged is yellow or white in the beginning, but in severe conditions it develops into a stage where the discharge is like pus mixed with a little blood. If this condition continues for long, it will develop into a chronic condition and the discharge will increase and the patient will suffer from anemia, constipation, lack of appetite, and irregular menstruation. In this state, it will be hard to conceive.

Treatment

Step One: Apply needle to SP-6 and LV-3.

Step Two: Apply needle to GV-4, BL-23, BL-27, BL-31, BL-32, BL-33, and BL-34, and continue with indirect moxa to all the points. If the patient is "overcooled," apply 5 direct moxa (red bean size) to BL-23.

Step Three: Apply needle to GB-26. If the condition is severe, apply 5 direct moxa (red bean size) after needling.

Step Four: Apply needle to CV-4 and CV-3. If the patient is "overcooled," apply 5 direct moxa (red bean size). If the leukorrhea is due to gonorrhea, apply 7 direct moxa (red or yellow bean size) to CV-3.

Prognosis: About ten treatments will suffice.

Prescription for Leukorrhea	
Step One	Boil one lb. of conch body, cut in small pieces, in six cups water.
Step Two	Boil down to one cup of liquid.
Step Three	While the conch is cooking, put 0.1 to 0.2 oz. of young antler of deer in a cup. When the conch liquid has been sufficiently reduced, pour it over the young deer antler and allow the mixture to cool slightly. Take one to three times.

Cancer of the Uterus

Cancer may occur in three different parts of the uterus: in the body of the uterus, in the neck of the uterus, or at the opening of the uterus to the vagina. Cancer in the body of the uterus is the most rare.

Causes: The cause of cancer is uncertain, but the disease occurs most often in elderly women. Cancer in the neck or cervix of the uterus usually occurs between the ages of 35 and 50; in the body of the uterus usually after 50 years of age. It is very rare among women under 20, and most women who develop cancer in the neck of the uterus have had children.

Symptoms: Cancer in its beginning stages is undetectable. As it develops, the first sign of its presence will be hemorrhage of the uterus. This appears early in the condition; as the condition becomes more advanced, the hemorrhage ceases.

The second sign of uterine cancer is vaginal discharge, which in the early stages is watery. As it develops, the discharge appears like pus mixed with blood.

The third sign is the pain, which is caused by the tumor's contact with adjacent organs. There will be slight pain at first in the ilium, the sacrum, and the lumbar region, developing into intense, piercing and tearing pain radiating down both legs. The fourth sign is the growing weakness of the patient, accompanied by loss of appetite, vomiting, pallor of the face and lips, loss of weight, and listlessness.

Treatment

Step One: Apply needle to SP-6, SP-9, and SP-10.

Step Two: Apply needle to CV-6, CV-4, CV-3, and CV-2.

Step Three: Apply needle to BL-23, BL-31, BL-32, BL-33, and BL-34.

Step Four: Apply needle to the lumps below the umbilicus (if these can be felt, which is sometimes possible in the case of cancer in the body of the uterus), or apply a long needle to the very painful spot or spots caused by the cancer. Follow by burning 3 moxa (one square inch in size) on the handle of the needle.

Step Five: If the cancer is in the neck of the uterus, apply 5 to 7 direct moxa (red bean size) to CV-3, CV-2, BL-33, and BL-34. Treat one point each day, returning to the first point on the fifth day and repeating the cycle.

Step Six: If the cancer is in the body of the uterus, on the first day apply 5 direct moxa (red bean size) to CV-4 and CV-3. On the second day, apply to BL-32 and BL-33. Continue alternating these points in this manner throughout the daily treatments.

Step Seven: If there is pain in the loins, apply 5 direct moxa (green bean size) to GB-26.

Step Eight: Apply 14 direct moxa (red bean size) to *Pee Gun* on both sides.

Note: When applying direct moxa in the fifth or sixth steps, continue with daily needle application as indicated in the **Steps One** through **Four**, including moxa on the handle of the needle.

Prognosis: In the first stage, ten to twenty treatments.

If the cancer has reached the stage where it has broken and caused the uterus to decay; if the pain is not relieved after needle and moxa application; or when surgery or a biopsy has been performed (this will cause the cancer to spread quickly), the cancer cannot be cured.

Prolapse of the Uterus

Causes: During childbirth, the mother has overstrained the abdominal muscles; after childbirth, the mother has been very angry, has not rested enough before resuming normal work activities, has had sexual intercourse in some abnormal manner, or has sat or laid down on some wet spot.

Symptoms: The uterus falls, and there is the sensation of having an object in the vagina.

Treatment

Step One: Apply needle to HT-8.

Step Two: Apply needle to SP-6, SP-9, and LV-1, and continue with 3 direct moxa (1/2 rice grain size) to LV-1.

Step Three: Apply needle to ST-25, CV-6, CV-4, and ST-29.

Step Four: Apply indirect moxa with ginger, or 5 direct moxa (red bean size) to GV-20 and/or GB-26.

Special Note: After treatment, the patient should lie in bed for several days. This will greatly assist the uterus in reverting back to its normal position.

Prognosis: In the early stages or mild conditions, two or three treatments will suffice. In chronic conditions, seven to ten treatments will effect recovery.

Ovaritis
— Inflammation of the Ovaries —

Causes: Puerperal fever; inflammation of the uterus; inflammation of the mucus membrane outside the uterus; leukorrhea; catarrh of the vagina.

Symptoms: Swelling and pain in the abdomen, and on the two sides below the level of the umbilicus. The pain comes on after the menstrual period. Pain increases on pressure. The patient has a fever and a feeling of chill. By vaginal or rectal examination, the ovaries are found to be enlarged. If the inflammation has subsided, the ovaries diminish in size in a few days. If the condition becomes severe, pus will exude from the ovaries and come out through the vagina, rectum or bladder. The patient suffers from constipation, poor appetite, and insomnia.

Treatment

Step One: Apply needle to LI-4.

Step Two: Apply needle to SP-9, SP-6, LV-1, and SP-10.

Step Three: Apply 3 direct moxa (sesame seed size) to LV-1, and 7 direct moxa (1/2 rice grain size) to XT-1 *(Tu Yin)*.

Step Four: Apply needle to ST-25 and ST-29.

Step Five: Apply indirect moxa to ST-29 and to the painful region.

Prognosis: About three to five treatments will suffice.

Difficulty in Childbirth
— Dystocia —

Causes: The fetus is positioned in the uterus improperly; lack of strength of the mother to press upon the uterus; the mother has not rested sufficiently or has overstrained herself so that she becomes too tired when the child is about to be born; the passage through which the baby will be born is too narrow.

Treatment

Step One: Apply 3 direct moxa (green bean size) to GV-20.

Step Two: Apply needle to LI-4.

Step Three: Apply needle to SP-6, LV-1, and BL-60.

Step Four: Apply needle to ST-25 and CV-4.

Step Five: Apply 7 direct moxa (1/2 rice grain size) to XT-1 *(Tu Yin)* and BL-67.

Prognosis: One treatment will suffice.

Special Note: If the pelvic outlet has been found to be too narrow for the baby to come out, Caesarian section should be performed by a medical doctor in the hospital.

Excessive Hemorrhage After Childbirth

Causes: Weakness of the mother's body.

Symptoms: Too much blood comes out from the uterus after childbirth, causing dizziness and fainting.

Treatment

Step One: Apply indirect moxa GV-20 and XF-3 *(Yin Tang).*

Step Two: Apply needle to TW-6.

Step Three: Apply needle to SP-6, ST-36. Apply 3 direct moxa (1/2 rice grain size) to LV-1 and SP-1.

Prognosis: About three treatments will suffice.

Special Note: If hemorrhage is from rupture of the major arteries, they must be packed or tied by a Western medical doctor.

Note: After childbirth, if the mother has paralysis of the four limbs, use the treatment for paralysis after a stroke.

Prescriptions for Women

For Paralysis after Confinement	
Step One	Fry about 8 oz of dove's feces, dry or fresh, in a clean pan until it is dry and produces a little smoke.
Step Two	Pour a little more than one cup of water over the cooked feces, and bring to a boil.
Step Three	Boil for a few minutes and pour the liquid through a filter. Give to the patient to drink.

Taken once a day for about three days the above prescription will help the patient feel much better, and may even effect a complete recovery.

For Emotional Upset and Dysmenorrhea		
Herb		Quantity
Chinese	Pharmaceutical Name	
1. 當歸	*Radix Angelica Sinensis*	9 grams
2. 白芍	*Radix Paeonia Lactiflora*	9 grams
3. 柴胡	*Radix Bupleuri*	9 grams
4. 雲苓	*Sclerotium Poriae*	12 grams
5. 白術	*Rhizoma Atractylodis Macrocephalae*	9 grams
6. 炙草	*Radix Glycyrrhizae*	3 grams
7. 生薑	*Radix Zingiberis*	2 pieces
8. 薄荷	*Herba Menthae*	2 grams
9. 丹皮	*Radix Moutan*	9 grams
10. 枝子炭	*Fructus Gardeniae*	9 grams

For emotional upset and bad temper, use herbs #1 to #8; for menstrual irregularities, especially irregular and excessive menstruation, use the entire prescription. Boil the herbs in 3 to 3 1/2 cups of water, until 1 cup remains. Allow to cool slightly, and drink in one dose.

For Menstrual Headache, Dizziness, Cramping in the Abdomen and/or Irregular Menses

Herb		Quantity
Chinese	Pharmaceutical Name	
酒黃芩	*Radix Scutelariae*	12 grams
春砂仁	*Fructus Amomi Villosi*	4.5 grams
白朮	*Rhizoma Atractylodis Macrocephalae*	12 grams
川芎	*Rhizoma Ligustici*	12 grams
雲苓	*Sclerotium Poriae*	12 grams
製香付	*Rhizoma Cyperi*	15 grams
益母草	*Herba Leonuri*	30 grams
續斷	*Radix Dipsaci Japonicae*	15 grams
台烏	*Radix Linderae*	24 grams
製玄胡	*Tuber Corydalis*	*12 grams*
黨參	*Radix Codonopsis*	12 grams
當歸	*Radix Angelica Sinensis*	24 grams
白芷	*Radix Angelica*	15 grams
陳皮	*Pericarpium Citri Reticulatae*	9 grams
丹參	*Radix Salvia Miltiorrhizae*	15 grams
熟地	*Radix Rehmanniae*	24 grams
屈金	*Tuber Curcumae Aromaticae*	9 grams
木香	*Radix Muhsiang*	9 grams
粉甘草	*Radix Glycyrrhizae*	6 grams

Grind the herbs into a fine powder, mix with good honey, and make into pills. Chew 1/2 oz. as gum, or swallow with warm water for each dose, once a day. To further increase its effectiveness, take with chicken soup.

The traditional Chinese pharmacist uses the *Ch'ien* (錢) (equal to approximately 3 grams) as the basic unit for weighing herbs in prescriptions.

For Anemia and Dizziness from Post-Partum Hemorrhage		
Herb		Quantity
Chinese	Pharmaceutical Name	
高麗參	*Panax Ginseng*	9 grams
黃芪	*Radix Astragali*	60 grams
當歸身	*Radix Angelicae Sinensis*	12 grams

The above prescription should be used after confinement, in cases where too much bleeding has caused anemia and dizziness. Boil the herbs in 4 cups of water until one cup of water remains. Allow to cool slightly before drinking. Take once a day, for about three days, to help supplement the blood.

Fright or Crying at Night

Causes: This is common among children under 8 years of age who are physically weak, who have eaten too much before going to bed, who are suffering from worms in the intestines or are affected by exciting stories or pictures.

Symptoms: During the night, the child suddenly cries and wakes up in fright, clinging to his or her parents. After 10 to 20 minutes the child calms down and is off to sleep again, or may cry for several hours without ceasing. Next morning the child will not be able to recall anything. This will continue every night or every other night.

Treatment

This treatment may be administered at the time of the episode, or the next day.

Step One: Apply 3 direct moxa (1/2 rice grain size) or indirect moxa with ginger to GV-20.

Step Two: Apply needle to PC-5 and HT-7.

Step Three: If the child's body is ''overheated,'' do not apply moxa to GV-20; instead, apply needle to PC-9 and draw out a few drops of blood.

Prognosis: Two or three treatments will suffice.

Chronic Lack of Appetite in Children

Causes: The milk from the bottle, or the entire diet, is unsuitable; overeating; use of dirty eating utensils; premature birth; anemia in childhood; worm infestation.

Symptoms: The face is pale and the muscles of the whole body are emaciated; the child has no desire to eat, the abdomen is distended and the urine is of a deep yellow color; the feces are always loose; the child scratches his hands, face, and nose, is constantly crying, and has a slight fever.

Special Diagnosis: Examine the palm of the child's hand and look at the fingers. One or more red or yellow spots in the XFi-1 *(Sze Fung)* points (at the middle crease of the four fingers, thumb excluded) indicates that the child is suffering from the illness.

Treatment

Step One: Use a triangular needle on each of the middle creases of the four fingers to the yellow or red spots. Press out the glue-like or gummy liquid from the spots. The needle should go no deeper than about 0.1″. One treatment may be insufficient and it may require 2 or 3 treatments until the glue has been extracted from the fingers.

Step Two: Apply triangular needle to HT-8. In some cases, the glue-like liquid will be found in this point. If so, press it out in the same manner as explained above.

Step Three: Apply needle to LI-4 and PC-6.

Step Four: Apply needle to ST-36 and CV-12. Alternatively, apply 3 direct moxa (green bean size) to these 2 points.

Prognosis: Two or three treatments will suffice.

Special Note: Do not apply triangular needle to exactly the same spot each time; apply at a slightly different spot with each treatment.

Tetany in a Newborn Baby

Causes: Tetanus infection of the newborn baby's umbilicus. Infection may be from the hands of the nurse or from the baby's bandage, or from the medical powder applied to the umbilicus. The germs remain in the umbilicus and excrete some poison which may injure the spinal cord or the medulla oblongata, and cause cramp in the whole body of the baby.

Symptoms: The first sign is that the baby finds it difficult to suck because of lockjaw. In the early stages, the lockjaw occurs intermittently, repeating after a few minutes. Gradually, the episodes of lockjaw become more frequent until finally the baby's jaw is locked completely. The cramp eventually extends beyond the jaw, and envelopes the entire face, the neck, the head and the back. The child will then bend the head backwards. Finally, the cramp will go down to the muscles of the chest and the baby will find it difficult to breathe. With lack of oxygen, the baby's muscles will show a bluish color through the skin. The cramp then reaches down to the intestines and the baby will stop breathing and will die. Just before death, the fever will reach 42 °C.

Treatment

• ***Treatment A for Tetany:***

There is a color line that goes up from the umbilicus in the direction of the sternum. If this line (which is not a vein) reaches the sternum, the baby cannot be saved. However, if the line has not reached the sternum, apply direct moxa (red bean size) to the top of the line. The line will come down a little at once. As soon as the line stops coming down any further, apply direct moxa again to the top of this line in its new position. This will then bring the line down lower. Continue to apply moxa until the line drops right down onto the umbilicus. Then apply 7 moxa on the umbilicus. This will cure the condition completely.

Some small white spots may be found on the baby's gums after the treatment. These white spots must be broken by rubbing with the finger wrapped in clean cotton wool. This procedure must follow the direct moxa treatment described above.

• *Treatment B for Tetany:*

Fill the umbilicus with salt, cover with a piece of ginger and apply moxa on the ginger (yellow bean size). Continue until the baby has recovered.

Methods **A** and **B** may be combined or used separately.

Prognosis: One or two treatments will bring about recovery.

Convulsions in Children

Causes: Fright in the daytime followed by fever; overeating and being unable to digest food; weakness of the body during dentition; inflammation of the ear with discharge.

Symptoms: This illness may come on quite suddenly, without warning and without signs and symptoms. More often, though, before the illness develops, the child will be unhappy and grind the teeth at night. Just before its onset, there will be a little cramp in the right hand, which gradually spreads to the entire body. This cramp will gradually loosen, but will continue with short spasms in the arms and legs. During the cramp attack there will be paralysis of the face, and the head will bend backwards. If the cramp subsides, the child may fall asleep again. In serious conditions, the attacks of cramp come on again and after a few hours. If this condition goes on for many days in this manner, the child will die. If the cramp is on only one side of the body, when it ceases and the child awakens there will be paralysis on this side of the body. During the attack, the child invariably has a high fever. Convulsions that occur only occasionally are rarely fatal.

Treatment

Step One: Apply needle to GV-26 and triangular or thick needle to XF-3 *(Yin Tang)*. Obtain a strong stimulus from XF-3.

Step Two: Apply needle to LI-4 and triangular needle to LU-11. Draw out a few drops of blood from LU-11.

Step Three: Apply triangular needle to SP-1 and obtain a strong stimulus.

Step Four: Apply thick needle to KI-1.

Step Five: Apply needle to BL-54 and BL-57, and obtain a strong stimulus from these two points.

Step Six: Apply needle to LI-11, GV-14, and CV-12.

Step Seven: If the condition is severe and the patient is in a severe state of body cramp, and is still unconscious, after applying the above 6 steps apply 3 to 5 direct moxa (red bean size) to GV-20, XF-3, and GV-24.

Step Eight: If, after applying the first six steps the patient is still stiff with cramp, apply 3 to 5 direct moxa (red bean size) to KI-1.

Step Nine: If the patient suffers from convulsions several times a month or several times a year, and if it is found that after acupuncture treatment he or she immediately recovers, it will still be necessary to apply 5 direct moxa (red bean size) to XF-3, KI-1, and CV-12. Apply direct moxa to the 3 points, one point daily in the order in which they are listed. If the patient can stand it, it is good to apply to all the 3 points in one day at one treatment.

Special Note: In mild conditions, the first step alone, or the last and the second steps, or the first three steps may suffice, and no further treatment is required. To avoid scarring the face, direct moxa on XF-3 should be avoided unless absolutely necessary.

Prognosis: In acute conditions, one treatment will suffice. In chronic conditions, three treatments will probably suffice.

Prescriptions for Children's Problems

For Extremely High Fever		
Herb		Quantity
Chinese	Pharmaceutical Name	
勾籐	*Ramulus et Uncus Uncariae*	1.6 grams
蟬退	*Peristracum Cicadae*	1.6 grams
羌活	*Radix Notopterygii*	1.6 grams
木通	*Caulis Mutung*	1.6 grams
枝子	*Fructus Gardeniae*	1.6 grams
杏仁	*Semen Pruni Armeniacae*	1.6 grams
甘草	*Radix Glycyrrhizae*	1.6 grams
防風	*Herba Ledebouriellae*	1.6 grams
京芥	*Herba Schizonepetae*	1.6 grams
薄荷	*Herba Menthae*	1.6 gram
山渣	*Fructus Crataegi et Preparatum*	3 grams
麥芽	*Fructus Hordei vel Tritici Germinatus*	3 grams
殭蠶	*Bombyx Mori L.*	6 grams
全蝎	*Buthus (Scorpion)*	6 grams

The above prescription is effective for bringing down a fever in a child whose fever cannot be brought down with medication. Boil the herbs in 2 cups of water until less than 1 cup remains, divide into three doses, and take throughout the day after the convulsions have ceased.

For Phlegm in the Throat, Pinworms in the Anus, and/or Inflammation and Swelling of the Knee		
Herb		Quantity
Chinese	Pharmaceutical Name	
硃砂	*Cinnabaris*	6 grams
天南星	*Tuber Arisaematis*	9 grams
神麯	*Massa Fermentata*	9 grams
巴豆霜	*Semen Tiglii*	6 grams
大黃	*Rhizoma Rhei*	6 grams

Mix the above herbs and grind to a fine powder. For removing phlegm, add a teaspoonful of sugar in 1/2 cup of hot water, mix in a pinch of the herb powder (somewhat less than a 1 mm. heap), and drink in one dose. This prescription will cause one or two loose bowel movements.

The traditional Chinese pharmacist uses the *Ch'ien* (錢) (equal to approximately 3 grams) as the basic unit for weighing herbs in prescriptions.

Severe Vomiting and Diarrhea in a Baby (Summer Diarrhea)

Causes: The baby is receiving bottled milk which is too thick or otherwise unsuitable; the baby has been given food it cannot digest. This illness most often occurs during the summer months, particularly in very hot, humid weather.

Symptoms: In the beginning, there is just a little vomiting after drinking milk, followed by frequent stools. In the early stages, the feces have a yellowish color, later becoming more and more watery. The smell of the feces at this stage is offensive, but as it becomes more watery the smell lessens. The baby develops a fever. With the onset of this illness the baby appears tired and weak, the eyes sink in, the face becomes emaciated and the fontanel that has not yet closed sinks slightly. The skin has an ashen white color. In the early stages, the baby is uncomfortable and restless and cannot sleep. When the disease has developed, the child is so weak that it hardly moves. In the beginning, the baby's tongue is coated, but later it becomes dry and red, and the baby is very thirsty. The pulse is rapid but very weak, and in serious conditions sometimes cannot be felt at all. Ocassionaly, the pulse is irregular. In some cases, the baby becomes unconscious and develops a high fever, dying within 24 hours.

Treatment

Step One: Apply thick needle to GV-26 and XF-3 *(Yin Tang).*

Step Two: Apply needle to LI-4 and PC-6.

Step Three: Apply needle to ST-36.

Step Four: Apply needle to CV-12, ST-25, CV-6, and CV-4.

Step Five: Apply indirect moxa with ginger or with instrument to XF-3, GV-20, and GV-14.

Step Six: Apply indirect moxa to CV-12, CV-8, ST-25, CV-6, and CV-4.

Step Seven: In severe conditions, the child's eyes become fixed, and foam may come from the mouth. This indicates that the child is dying and that, in fact, it may die within half an hour. In this condition, immediately apply 5 direct moxa (red bean size) to both sides of LV-13. This may save the child.

Prognosis: One to two treatments should suffice. In severe conditions, three or four treatments will bring about recovery. The child's diet *must* be modified, eliminating cold foods and drinks, and raw vegetable and fruits for a few days.

Meningitis

Causes: Germs of meningitis. The disease usually comes on in the winter or spring, and stronger children are more susceptible to it. The germs enter the body through the mouth or the nose.

Symptoms: In some cases, with the onset of the illness there will be such signs as a two or three day period of unusual unhappiness, with headache and pain in the upper back region and in the legs or arms. In most cases, however, the illness comes on suddenly with a high fever (over 40 °C), severe headache, and stiffness of the neck, with the head bending directly back. If you try to bend the head forwards, the child will suffer excruciating pain and cry out. The child is semi-conscious, and in some cases suffers from cramp of the body, enlargement of the pupils, closed eyelids, eyes fixed on one side, and paralysis of the facial nerves. If the disease occurs in a baby, the fontanel will become swollen.

Special Diagnosis: With high fever, delirium, stiffness of the neck, and the head bending backwards, the acupuncturist should press hard upon GV-26 and PC-9 with the fingernail. If the patient cries, the patient can be cured; if the patient does not cry, the patient cannot be cured.

Have the patient close his or her fist. If the patient is a boy, examine the left fist. If upon closing his fist, his thumb remains out, this indicates that he can easily be cured. If, upon closing his fist, he covers his thumb with his fingers, this is a clear indication that this case is difficult to cure.

If the patient is a girl, examine the right fist. If upon closing her fist, the patient covers her thumb with her fingers, the case will be easy to cure. If, upon closing her fist, her thumb remains sticking out, this case will be difficult to cure.

In both boys and girls, if, upon closing the fist, the thumb is placed between the forefinger and the middle finger and juts out between then, the case is hopeless.

Treatment

Step One: Apply needle to PC-6, SI-3, LI-11, and PC-3. After applying needle, draw a few drops of blood from vein near PC-3.

Step Two: Apply needle to ST-36, SP-9, GB-34, GB-39, BL-57, GB-30, GB-31, and BL-54. After applying needle to the BL-54, draw out a few drops of blood from the vein near this point. Finally, needle KI-1.

Step Three: Apply needle to GV-26, CV-24, GB-20, GV-16, and GV-20. After applying needle, use triangular needle to draw out a few drops of blood from GV-20. Continue by applying needle to ST-8, XF-2, and *Tai Yang*.

Step Four: Apply needle to CV-22, CV-13, CV-12, CV-10, and CV-6.

Step Five: Apply needle to BL-13, BL-23, GV-2, and GV-4.

Prognosis: Cure is only effective in 30 percent the meningitis cases. There is more hope in early treatment of the patient.

Prescription for Meningitis
Pound a fresh dandelion into pulp and apply to GV-20. This will prove to be very effective.

Polio

Acute Inflammation of the Anterior Horn Cells

Causes: Polio usually attacks children between the ages of one and four. The disease commences with a high fever, measles or scarlet fever. It can also start with a cold, external injury, a sudden fright, or during teething. It is understood now to be a caused by a virus.

Symptoms: This disease starts with chill and high fever between 39° and 40 °C. The baby will be unhappy, hateful, and anorexic. This will be followed by headaches, vomiting, sacral pain, and trembling in the four limbs. Semiconscious and unconscious states follow. Muscles become spastic and cramped. High fever may last for several hours or 2 to 3 days. Paralysis then ensues. Usually the left lower limb is affected, although some experience it on the right side or on all four limbs. The mildest form produces only facial paralysis. The muscle becomes emaciated on the paralyzed limb. Sensation is still present, but no movement is possible. The bladder functions normally.

Treatment

• ***For paralysis of the upper limbs:***

Apply needle to GB-21, LI-15, LI-11, LI-10, LI-4, and TW-5. For light ailments, use indirect moxa by instrument or ginger after needling. For severe conditions, use direct moxa or God's needle on the above points.

• ***For paralysis of the lower limbs:***

Apply needle to BL-54, GB-30, GB-34, GB-39, SP-9, SP-6, BL-60, KI-3, BL-23, and BL-31, BL-32, BL-33, BL-34. If both legs are paralyzed, treat points bilaterally; if one side, treat diseased side. Follow moxa indications as prescribed for four limbs, except BL-54.

• ***For facial paralysis: Follow the treatment under* Apoplexy, Condition III.**

Prognosis: For light ailments, seven to ten treatments are needed. For severe conditions, twenty to thirty. If the case is 1/2 to 1 year old, it is hard to say how many treatments would be needed.

Rheumatism in the Muscles

Causes: Catching cold frequently; constantly working in the water or in a mine; always sleeping on the ground or stone floor; external injury.

Symptoms: Pain in the affected muscle of the body, occasionally with cramp or swelling. The pain may last as little as a few hours or as long as a few weeks in acute conditions; in chronic conditions, the pain may continue for even longer. Rheumatism occurs more easily in the muscles of the shoulders, the neck, the upper back, and the lumbar region. This illness is very subject to changes of temperature, and often worsens with cold weather. Warm weather may bring some relief to the patient. Persons over 40 years of age are most susceptible.

Treatment

• ***Treatment of rheumatism in the upper part of the back***

Step One: Apply needle to GV-26, TW-3, and BL-54.

Step Two: Apply needle to BL-12, BL-38, and the center of the painful spot. After applying the needle, in mild conditions apply indirect moxa to the painful region; in severe or chronic conditions, apply 5-10 direct moxa (red bean size) or indirect moxa on the handle of the needle to the center of the painful region, on the most painful spot.

• ***Treatment of rheumatism in the muscles of the shoulder***

Step One: Apply needle to GB-21 and LI-15.

Step Two: Apply needle to LI-10 and TW-3.

Step Three: Apply needle to BL-12 and BL-38.

Step Four: Apply needle to the center of the most painful spot. In mild conditions, continue with indirect moxa. In severe conditions, apply 5 to 10 direct moxa (red bean size), or indirect moxa on the handle of the needle to the center of the painful region.

• *Treatment of rheumatism in the muscles of the neck (stiffness of the neck)*

Step One: Apply needle to SI-3.

Step Two: Apply needle to GB-20, GB-21, BL-10, GV-16, and XN-1 *(Pak Loh)*.

Step Three: Apply needle to GV-14 and BL-11. (For application to GV-14, use acrossing needle technique on the affected side.)

Step Four: Apply needle to the center of the painful region in the same manner as in the preceding case.

• *Treatment of lumbago*

Step One: Apply needle to BL-54 and GB-30.

Step Two: Apply needle to BL-23.

Step Three: Apply needle to the center of the painful region in the same manner as in the step above.

Step Four: If the pain in the lumbar region is very severe, apply 5 direct moxa (red bean size) to SP-2. (If the pain is in the left side of the lumbar region, apply to SP-2 of the left foot.)

Note: On the first treatment, after treating with the needle, search the muscle and see if there is any *Sha*. If there is, do *Gwa Sha*. Do not use moxa right away.

Prognosis: In mild conditions, 3 to 5 treatments will suffice. In chronic or very old conditions, over 10 treatments.

Arthritis

Neuralgia or Rheumatism in the Joints of the Body

Causes: Arthritis comes on suddenly, and results from external injury, anemia, from a bout of intense anger, or after an infectious disease.

Symptoms: This illness may occur in any joint of the body, although it occurs most commonly in the knee and hip joints. The pain is very severe, and will spread upwards and downwards. Sometimes the skin over the joint is reddish in color as a result of the rheumatism. Because of the pain in the joints, the patient may be unable to use his or her limbs. The patient desires to stretch out the affected limb. If this illness is allowed to continue for a long time, the muscles will atrophy.

Treatment

• ***Treatment of neuralgia or rheumatism in the shoulder joint***

Step One: Apply needle to LI-15, GB-21, LI-16, and LI-14.

Step Two: Apply indirect moxa to all the points of **Step One**.

Step Three: If the condition is severe, apply 3 direct moxa (red bean size) to LI-15.

Assistant Points: BL-12 and BL-38.

• ***Treatment of neuralgia or rheumatism in the elbow joint***

Step One: Apply needle to LU-5, PC-3, and LI-11.

Step Two: Apply indirect moxa to all the points of step one except LU-5.

Step Three: If there is a particularly painful spot in the region, in mild conditions, apply indirect moxa on the painful spot. In severe conditions, after needling apply 3 direct moxa (red bean size) to the painful spot.

If the pain is just on one elbow, treat the affected side only.

Assistant Points: PC-6, HT-3, TW-3, TW-2, and SI-8.

• ***Treatment of neuralgia or rheumatism in the wrist joint***

Step One: Apply needle to SI-4, LU-9, LI-5, TW-4, TW-5, and the spot where the pain is most severe. After this, in mild conditions, apply indirect moxa to the painful spot and the points close to it.

Step Two: Apply 5 to 7 direct moxa (red bean size) to the painful spots.

Assistant Points: SI-3 and HT-4.

• ***Treatment of neuralgia or rheumatism of the hip joint***

Step One: Apply needle to BL-54, GB-31, GB-30, and the most painful spot.

Step Two: Apply indirect moxa with instrument or by burning moxa on the handle of the needle to GB-30 and to the painful spot.

Assistant Points: Apply needle to BL-23 and 3 direct moxa (red bean size) to SP-2.

Note: In the above case, look for *sha* after needle treatment.

• ***Treatment of neuralgia or rheumatism in the knee joint***

Step One: Apply needle to GB-34, SP-9, BL-54, and XL-1 *(Shi Yan)*.

Step Two: Apply needle to BL-54, using a long needle, and let it penetrate 1 1/2 to 2 inches, until the needle touches the bone. The stimulus should be felt under the patella bone.

Step Three: Apply indirect moxa with instrument or by burning moxa on the handle of the needle at XL-1 *(Shi Yan)*, SP-9, and GB-34.

Assistant Points: ST-33, GB-31, LV-8, ST-36, GB-33, and GB-39.

• ***Treatment of neuralgia or rheumatism in the ankle joint***

Step One: Apply needle to KI-6, BL-60, KI-3, and BL-62.

Step Two: If the pain is in the front part of the joint, apply needle to SP-5, GB-40, and LV-4. If there is a particularly painful spot, apply the needle there, and then continue with indirect moxa with the instrument or by burning moxa on the handle of the needle.

Prognosis: In mild conditions, 1 to 3 treatments. In chronic or severe conditions, 7 to 10 or more treatments.

Numbness of the Deltoid Muscle

Causes: Numbness in the nerves of the shoulder; external injury to the shoulder; neuritis or rheumatism of the shoulder; illness affecting the spinal cord.

Symptoms: The patient finds it extremely difficult to raise the arms. This condition is divided into the following three symptom patterns:

Numbness in the Anterior Portion of the Deltoid: Here the patient will find it difficult to raise his or her arm in front and will be unable to touch the shoulder of the other arm.

Numbness in the Posterior Portion of the Deltoid: In this condition, the patient will be unable to place the hand on the affected side of his or her upper back.

Numbness in the Lateral Portion of the Deltoid: In this case, the patient will not be able to raise his or her arm to shoulder level.

Treatment

• *Treatment of Anterior Deltoid Numbness*

Step One: Apply needle to GB-21, LI-15, LI-11 and LI-4.

Step Two: Following step one, apply indirect moxa with the instrument or by burning moxa upon the needle, or direct moxa to GB-21 and LI-15.

• *Treatment of Posterior Deltoid Numbness*

Step One: Apply needle to LI-15, LI-14, LI-16, LU-5, and TW-3.

Step Two: Following step one, apply indirect moxa with the instrument or by burning moxa on handle of the needle, or direct moxa to LI-15, LI-16, and LI-14.

• *Treatment of Lateral Deltoid Numbness*

Step One: Apply needle to LI-15, PC-3, LI-11, LI-10 and LI-14.

Step Two: Following step one, apply indirect moxa with the instrument or by burning moxa on the handle of the needle, or direct moxa to LI-15 and LI-14.

Special Note: Sometimes the patient will suffer *both* posterior and anterior numbness, or *both* posterior and lateral numbness. In these cases, combine the treatments. After the treatment, palpate the area to discover any painful spots. Apply the needle there, and follow with moxa , either indirect or direct. If painful spot(s) cannot be found, assist the patient in gently raising his or her arm. The painful spot will then reveal itself. Treat the painful spot as directed.

Assistant Points: BL-12, BL-38, BL-10, GB-20, LU-1, LV-13, TW-6, and HT-3.

Prognosis: In acute and mild conditions, 3 to 5 treatments. In chronic or severe conditions, 10 or more treatments. Some cases are very difficult to cure.

Common Ailments of the Hand and Arm

• ***Pain in the whole arm, from the shoulder down to the hand***

Apply needle to LI-15, LI-14, LI-13, LI-11, and LI-10, and follow with indirect moxa to all points.

• ***Mild stiffness of the arm***

Apply needle to LI-11, LU-5, PC-3, and PC-7, and follow with indirect moxa to all the points.

• ***Weakness of the wrist joint***

Apply needle to SI-4, LU-9, LU-7, and follow with indirect moxa to all points, or direct moxa to SI-4, LI-5, and TW-4.

• ***Cold and pain in the whole arm***

Apply indirect moxa, God's needle, or direct moxa to GB-21, LI-15, LI-14, and LI-11. (Do not apply needle to any these points.) This is an ''overcooled'' condition. The most effective treatment is to treat GV-14 with moxa (red bean size).

• ***Cramp of the fingers***

Apply needle to LI-11, LI-10, PC-3, PC-5, PC-7, and LI-4, and follow with indirect moxa or God's needle to all the points, or direct moxa to PC-3 and PC-7.

• ***Pain in the fingers***

Apply needle to TW-5 and LU-11. Use a thick needle and obtain a strong stimulus from LU-11. No moxa is required. It is also effective to treat the 8 ghost points and follow with indirect moxa.

• *Boil or abscess on the finger (''snake's head boil'') accompanied by pus and severe pain*

If not cured, this condition can destroy the finger joint. Apply needle to LI-11 on both arms, LI-10 on the arm with the affected finger, PC-7, and TW-5. If any of these points are close to the finger affected, apply the needle to them as well. If the boil has just begun and is still without pus, apply indirect moxa with ginger on the boil. If there is some pus inside, or the condition has developed into an abscess or ulcer, or has opened, apply 3-5 direct moxa (red bean size) to LI-11 of both arms.

• *Pain in the Palmar Aspect of the Arm*

Apply needle to LU-9 and PC-3. Indirect moxa will also be helpful.

• *Cramp of the elbow joint*

Apply needle to LU-5, PC-3, LI-11, PC-5, PC-7, and SI-3. After this apply God's needle to the elbow region. For chronic cases, apply 5 direct moxa to PC-3 and PC-7.

• *Condition where the patient cannot close the fist and/or cannot bend the elbow.*

Apply needle to LI-11, LU-5, PC-3, LI-10, TW-5, and TW-3. After this, apply indirect moxa or God's needle to these points.

• *Numbness in the tips of the fingers*

Apply needle to LI-4, PC-7, SI-4, LU-5, TW-6, and 8 ghost points or the well points without bleeding them, as well as 7 green-bean size moxa on PC-7.

Parkinson's Disease

Causes: The true cause of Parkinson's disease is not known, but it may develop as the sequelae of influenza, syphilis, or an external injury. This disease occurs in persons over 40 years of age, and is more common in men than in women. The disease starts with lack of energy and weakness of the heart.

Symptoms: Parkinson's disease comes on very gradually, and in the beginning there are no symptoms. In most cases, it starts with shaking of the right hand and gradually develops in the other hand and the legs, Finally, a time comes when the entire body, including the head and mouth, shake tremulously. In milder cases, the shaking ceases when the patient writes or does something with the hands. If the patient is greatly excited or angry, the shaking will be more severe, but when the patient falls asleep the shaking will cease. The muscles will stiffen and the eyes become very fixed with little movement of the eyes. The patient walks with small, quick steps and, without his or her hand to assist, cannot stop and continues walking with small quick, steps. The patient perspires and has a mild fever, tears flow from the eyes, and saliva from the mouth.

Treatment

Step One: Apply 5 direct moxa (red bean size) to HT-3 and ST-33, and 7 moxa on GV-14.

Step Two: **For the arm:** Apply needle to LI-15, LI-11, LU-5, PC-3, and LI-4.

Step Three: **For the leg:** Apply needle to GB-30, GB-31, GB-34, GB-39 and SP-6, BL-60, KI-3, and BL-54.

Special Note: If only one hand shakes, use only steps one and two. If the shaking develops so that it is in the leg and/or feet, use all three steps.

Prognosis: If the illness has shown itself for only 1/2 year, it can be easily cured; after 1/2 year, it is more difficult to cure; and if it is of several years duration it is extremely difficult to cure.

Sciatica

Causes: Sciatica (neuralgia of the sciatic nerve) is more common than neuralgia in other specific nerves of the body. It is caused by catching cold in the body; external injury to the leg or in the region of the sciatic nerve; a carbuncle in the region of the sciatic nerve; pregnancy; constipation; from any disease in the lumbar vertebrae; or from diabetes, syphilis, rheumatism, inflammation of the spinal cord, or neuritis of the sciatic nerve.

Symptoms: Pain in the buttock which may extend down to the knee and gradually down to the ankle bone. The pain is always particularly severe at night. If the sciatica is not cured within 2 or 3 months, the muscles of the leg will atrophy.

Treatment

Step One: Apply needle to GV-26 and BL-54.

Step Two: Apply needle to BL-23 on the affected side, and continue with indirect moxa on the same points. If the condition is severe, apply 5 direct moxa (red bean size) to BL-23.

Step Three: Apply needle to GB-30 and GB-31, and continue with indirect moxa. If the condition is severe, apply 5 direct moxa (red bean size) to these 2 points.

Step Four: Apply needle to GB-34, GB-39, and BL-60. In severe cases, 5 direct moxa should be applied to GB-34, GB-39, and BL-60. After this, the pain will not come back again.

Step Five: If the condition is very severe, apply 3 direct moxa (red bean size) to SP-2.

Step Six: If there is any particularly painful spot, apply the needle to the spot and continue with indirect moxa , moxa on the handle of the needle, or direct moxa to the painful spot.

Note: Apply the needle only to the affected side of the body.

Assistant Points:BL-25, BL-28, BL-31, BL-32, BL-33, BL-34, GV-2, GB-38, GV-1, BL-30, SP-9, and BL-57.

Prognosis: In mild conditions, 2 to 4 treatments will bring about recovery. In severe conditions, over 10 treatments are necessary.

Diseases in the Leg and Foot

• *Numbness of the leg and foot*

Step One: Apply needle to GV-2, GB-30, GB-31, GB-34, SP-9, ST-36, SP-6, GB-39, KI-3, and BL-60.

Step Two: Follow **Step One** with indirect moxa or God's needle to all the points of that step.

Step Three: Apply 3 direct moxa (1/2 rice grain size) to BL-67, and 5 direct moxa (red-bean size) on GB-31.

Prognosis: Length of treatment depends upon condition of patient.

• *Cramp of the leg with inability to stretch out the leg*

Step One: Apply needle to BL-23, and in mild conditions continue with indirect moxa or God's needle to BL-23. In severe conditions, apply 7 direct moxa (red bean size) to BL-23.

Step Two: Apply needle to BL-31, BL-32, BL-33, BL-34, and continue with indirect moxa or God's needle to these points.

Step Three: Apply needle to BL-54, GB-31, GB-34, GB-38, and BL-57. Continue with indirect moxa or God's needle to same points; also moxa 5 times to KI-1 and BL-57.

Prognosis: Length of treatment depends on patient's condition.

• *Icy cold feet in winter:*

Step One: Apply 10 direct moxa (red bean size) to GV-4.

Step Two: Apply 7 direct moxa (red bean size) to BL-23

Step Three: Apply 5 direct moxa (red bean size) to ST-36. If the patient is afraid of pain from direct moxa, use the God's needle or divide in 3 treatments.

Step Four: Apply 5-10 direct moxa (red-bean size) to GV-3.

Prognosis: With direct moxa, 7 daily treatments will suffice. With God's needle, daily treatment for 3 weeks or more will be necessary.

• ***Cramp in the calf or in the sole of the foot***

Apply needle to BL-57 and continue with indirect moxa. If the case is chronic or severe apply 5 direct moxa (red bean size) to BL-57.

• ***Cramp in the sole of the foot***

Apply needle to KI-1, and in mild conditions continue with 7 direct moxa (green bean size), flicking the moxa off as soon as the patient feels pain. In chronic or severe conditions, after applying the needle to KI-1, the 7 direct moxa should be burned on the point without flicking them off.

• ***Weak knees, causing difficulty standing or walking***

Step One: Apply needle to BL-54 as deep as possible and obtain the stimulus in the back of the patella bone.

Step Two: Apply needle to ST-33, ST-36, and to the outer and inner XL-1 (Eyes of Knee). Continue with indirect moxa or God's needle, or moxa on the handle of the needle to both XL-1. If the condition is severe or chronic, apply 7 direct moxa (red bean size) to both XL-1, and also 7 direct moxa (green bean size) to *Hok Deng* (XL-2).

• ***Pain in the Heel***

Step One: Apply needle to KI-8 and obtain stimulus down to the heel.

Step Two: Apply needle to, KI-7, KI-3, KI-5, and KI-6. If the pain ceases after applying needle to KI-8 and KI-7, it is unnecessary to apply to KI-6, KI-5, and KI-3.

Step Three: If the condition is chronic, and after applying the needle to the points of the second step the pain ceases but returns again on the following day, apply 5 direct moxa (green bean size) to KI-8 and KI-7. Continue with the direct moxa daily for 2 days, or apply 7 direct moxa to the most painful spot of the heel instead of on KI-7 and KI-8.

Prognosis: In mild or acute conditions, one treatment. In chronic conditions, three treatments should suffice.

Acute Inflammation of the Synovial Fluid of the Knee

Causes: External injury or blow to the knee; inflammation in some other part of the body being diverted to the knee; sequelae of gonorrhea or syphilis; catching cold with a high fever in the whole body.

Symptoms: The principal sign is swelling of the knee, with pain, inflammation and reddish color of the skin of the knee. As the liquid in the knee accumulates, the knee will become more swollen. Upon palpation of the side of the knee, the patella will seem to float as if it were on top of the knee. If the knee is moved it will be painful. Usually the patient does not have a high fever, although there may be mild fever in some cases.

Treatment

Step One: Apply needle to SP-9, GB-34, SP-10, and ST-33.

Step Two: Apply needle to ST-36, LV-8, SP-6, and GB-39.

Step Three: Apply needle to BL-54 as deeply as possible and obtain the stimulus at the back of the patella bone.

Step Four: Apply needle to XL-1 *(Shi Yan)* as deeply as possible and continue with 3 moxa burned on the handle of the needle. In severe conditions, apply 7 direct moxa (red or yellow bean size) to XL-1. After treating XL-1, apply 5 direct moxa each day to one of the following pairs of points, one pair each day: ST-33 and SP-10, and SP-9 and GB-34.

Prognosis: In mild conditions, about 10 treatments. In severe or chronic conditions, 30 or more treatments.

Beri-Beri

Causes: Vitamin B deficiency.

Symptoms: Beri-beri occurs as three distinct symptom patterns: *dry beri-beri*, *wet beri-beri*, and *acute beri-beri*.

Dry beri-beri: The whole body is affected with neuritis, and the muscles gradually become thinner and small. There is great weakness in the legs, and the patient is hardly able to walk.

Wet beri-beri: The first sign is that the leg is swollen as in dropsy. The neuritis is milder than in dry beri-beri. When walking, the patient feels that the legs are very heavy. In both dry and wet beri-beri the heart is very weak and there is the feeling of something pressing on the chest (like mild angina pectoris).

Acute beri-beri: In this condition, there is no neuritis in the legs, but only the heavy pressing feeling upon the heart. The patient may faint at any time as the heart is very weakened. If the patient faints, the condition is dangerous and death may occur easily.

In the early stages of the first two types of beri-beri, the patient feels in an abnormal state, and feels heaviness in the legs, gradually loses appetite, suffers from heart palpitations, and fast and short breath. However, when busy with work the patient does not notice this condition. As time goes on, the numbness in the legs is noticed as is the gradual swelling or weakening of the leg muscles. In acute beri-beri, the heart suddenly shows its weakness, and in this weakened condition, death approaches rapidly.

Treatment

• ***Treatment of Dry Beri-Beri***

Step One: Apply needle followed by 3 direct moxa (green bean size) to GB-31.

Step Two: Apply needle to SP-9, GB-34, ST-36, SP-6, GB-39, KI-3, BL-60, BL-67, and KI-1. Directly after, apply indirect moxa to all the points of step two until skin is a reddish color.

• *Treatment for Wet Beri-Beri*

Step One: Apply needle followed by 3 direct moxa (green bean size) to GB-31.

Step Two: Apply needle to ST-36, SP-6, GB-39, and BL-57. Continue with indirect moxa to all points until the skin is a reddish color.

• *Treatment Acute Beri-Beri*

Step One: Apply needle followed by 3-5 direct moxa (green bean size) to GB-31. If the patient is actually in a fainting spell at the time of treatment, do not bother with the needle, but apply 5-10 direct moxa (green bean size) immediately to GB-31. The patient will regain consciousness immediately.

Step Two: Apply needle to ST-36, SP-6, and GB-39, and continue with indirect moxa to all points of step two until the skin is a reddish color.

Prognosis: For dry beri-beri, 7 treatments; for wet beri-beri, 3 treatments; for acute beri-beri, 3 treatments will be required.

Malaria

Causes: Malaria germs enter the body through bites of the Anopheles mosquito.

Symptoms: From 1 to 3 weeks after the initial infection, the patient feels very cold at first and shivers and then develops fever. The pulse is full (feels very strong, but is really not). There is great thirst and severe headache. After a few hours, the patient perspires and the fever lessens. Some hours later, the temperature returns to normal or even becomes subnormal.

In some cases, the attacks are daily; in others, the attacks come every second or third day. The attacks come at the same time each day. If this condition lasts for long, the patient's spleen will become swollen. There is one often fatal type of malaria in which there is not much of a chill, the fever is very high, and the patient suffers from diarrhea, vomiting, fainting, and delirium, with possible jaundice, ulcers in the liver, and extreme weakness of the body.

Treatment

• ***Treatment Method A, when the attacks are daily, every other day or every third day***:

Step One: Apply needle to GV-14 and continue with indirect moxa until the skin is reddish in color. If the condition is severe, apply 7 direct moxa (green bean size).

Step Two: Apply needle to PC-5 and SI-3. In mild conditions, apply indirect moxa to these two points until the skin has changed to a reddish color. In severe or chronic conditions, apply 3 direct moxa (green or red bean size). The above treatment should be done three hours before the attack starts.

• ***Treatment Method B, during rigor (i.e., while the patient is experiencing an attack of severe chills or high fever):***

Apply needle to BL-38 or all the well points on the fingers of both hands. This will stop the fever and the severe cold at once. Then ask the patient at what time the attack commenced. On the next day, exactly three hours before the expected attack, apply the *Treatment Method A*, above.

• ***Treatment Method C, for chronic malaria that has lasted for 2 or 3 years***:

Apply *Treatment Method A*. Then apply 7 direct moxa (red bean size) to BL-20. Three daily treatments are necessary.

• ***Treatment Method D, for chronic malaria that has lasted 1 to 3 years, and when the patient's spleen has swelled up and enlarged:***

Apply *Treatment Methods A* and *C*. Apply needle to LV-13 on the left side of the body only, as well as BL-20 and ST-25 on the left side. Apply needle to ST-36 on both legs. After this, on the first day apply 14 direct moxa (yellow bean size) to *Pee Gun*. On the 2nd day apply 7 direct moxa (red bean size) to BL-20 instead of *Pee Gun* on the left side only, and continue apply needle to LV-13, BL-20, ST-25, on the left side and direct moxa to BL-20 for three daily treatments. On the 5th day, after applying needle to LV-13, BL-20, ST-25, apply 5 direct moxa (red bean size) to LV-13. Each time apply needle to ST-36 also. Continue with this procedure for 3 daily treatments. After this (7 days since the first day's treatment) if the spleen has not become normal, repeat the whole treatment over again.

• ***Treatment Method E, malaria with delirium and very high fever, no cold feeling and loss of consciousness:***

Use *Treatment Methods A* and *B*, including all the well points of the fingers of both hands, using only the needle. Do not use moxa at all. For each point of the fingers use the triangular needle and draw out a few drops of blood.

Prognosis: In mild conditions, 1 to 3 treatments will suffice. In severe or chronic conditions, about 5 treatments. In case of swollen spleen, 10 to 20 treatments.

Special Note: After recovery, for a half a month the patient must avoid eating cold or iced foods or drinks, and avoid raw vegetables and fruits. This will keep the body in a warm condition, the germs of malaria will all die within the half month, and the illness will not return unless the patient is reinfected.

Influenza

Causes: Influenza virus, which chiefly attacks the bronchial tubes and the nasal passage. An infected person who coughs or sneezes will infect others. Persons of any age may be infected. After an attack of influenza, the patient is easily reinfected.

Symptoms: Within 1 to 3 days after infection, the patient has a cold feeling, with fever, headache, pain in the eyeballs, lumbar pain, and pain in the arms and legs. At the same time, the mucus membrane of the nasal and bronchial passages will be inflamed, and the patient will sneeze and cough frequently. It is difficult for the patient to expectorate the phlegm. The patient feels very weak. Sometimes there are nose bleeds, vomiting, and delirium. Sometimes the virus affects the stomach and the intestines, with pain in the abdomen accompanied by vomiting and diarrhea. Some patients may have their brain affected, and may be sleepless and delirious, with pain in all the joints in the arms and/or legs. Complications sometimes occur, the most common of which is pneumonia, which often brings about death. If the patient suffers from tuberculosis in the lungs, an attack of influenza will have severe effects. The virus weakens the patient's heart. Inflammation of the nose and discharge from the middle ear are common after an attack of influenza.

Treatment

Step One: Apply needle to LI-4 and BL-54.

Step Two: Apply needle to GB-20, GV-14, and BL-12.

If the condition is mild, the patient will perspire all over the body and the fever will drop almost immediately. In this case, nor further treatment is necessary.

Step Three: If after the 1st and 2nd steps, the patient still has a cold feeling in the back, apply indirect moxa to GV-14, GV-13, and BL-12 until the patient feels that the back has warmed up.

Step Four: If after the 1st and 2nd steps the patient still has a high fever, apply triangular needle to LU-11 and PC-9 and draw out a few drops of blood from each of these two points.

Step Five: If the patient has the feeling of something pressing upon the heart, apply needle to GB-21 penetrating 1 1/2", and obtain a stimulus down to the chest. If the patient suffers from heart palpitations, angina pectoris, or weakness of the heart, do not apply needle to GB-21, but apply needle to LV-14 and LU-1.

Step Six: If the patient suffers from a cough, apply needle to BL-13.

Step Seven: If the patient suffers from a headache, apply needle to ST-8.

Step Eight: If the patient suffers from a heavy feeling in the eyebrows, apply needle to BL-2 and TW-23.

Step Nine: If the patient vomits, apply needle to PC-6 and CV-12.

Step Ten: If the patient suffers from diarrhea, apply needle to ST-36, ST-25, and CV-4.

Step Eleven: If there is another disease accompanying the influenza, treat both diseases at the same time.

Assistant Points: GV-16, GV-13, BL-38, and LI-11.

Prognosis: 1 to 3 treatments will bring about recovery.

Prescriptions for Influenza

Prescription I for Influenza		
Herb		Quantity
Chinese	Pharmaceutical Name	
麻黃	*Herba Ephedra*	9 grams
桂枝	*Ramulus Cinnamomi*	9 grams
北杏仁	*Semen Pruni Armeniacae*	9 grams
炙甘草	*Radix Glycyrrhizae Preparata*	6 grams

This prescription is indicated for a flu accompanied by chill, headache, stiffness of neck, no perspiration, and when a floating pulse is found on both hands. Boil the herbs in 2 cups of water until less than 1 cup remains and drink while warm.

Prescription II for Influenza		
Herb		Quantity
Chinese	Pharmaceutical Name	
桂枝	*Ramulus Cinnamomi*	9 grams
白芍	*Radix Paeonia Alba*	9 grams
炙甘草	*Radix Glycyrrhizae Preparata*	6 grams
大棗	*Fructus Zizyphi Jujubae*	3 pieces
生薑	*Radix Zingiberis Recens*	2 slices

This prescription is recommended for a flu accompanied by chill, headache, and perspiration, and when a floating pulse is found on both wrists. Boil the herbs in 2 1/2 cups of water until 1 cup remains. Drink when warm.

Prescription III for Influenza		
Herb		Quantity
Chinese	Pharmaceutical Name	
銀花	*Flos Lonicerae*	9 grams
連喬	*Fructus Forsythiae*	9 grams
桔梗	*Radix Platycodi Grandiflori*	9 grams
淡竹葉	*Herba Gracilis*	9 grams
薄荷	*Herba Menthae*	1.5 grams
荊芥	*Herba seu Flos Schizonepetae Tenuifolia*	7.5 grams
淡豆鼓	*Semen Sojae Preparatum*	9 grams
牛蒡子	*Fructus Arctii Lappae*	9 grams
生甘草	*Radix Glycyrrhizae*	3 grams
蘆根	*Rhizoma Phragmatis Communis*	15 grams
神麴	*Massa Fermentata*	9 grams
花粉	*Radix Tricosanthis*	9 grams

When a flu is accompanied by a smooth and big pulse on the right wrist or on both wrists, this prescription is appropriate. Boil the herbs in 3 1/2 cups of water until 1 cup remains and drink when warm. After taking this prescription, the patient should lie in bed, covered with a blanket, to promote perspiration. After sweating, recovery will soon follow.

Prescription IV for Influenza		
Herb		Quantity
Chinese	Pharmaceutical Name	
北杏	*Semen Pruni Armeniacae*	9 grams
連喬	*Fructus Forsythiae*	9 grams
冬桑葉	*Folium Mori Alba*	9 grams
薄荷	*Herba Menthae*	2 grams
桔梗	*Radix Platycodi Grandiflori*	9 grams
甘菊花	*Herba Allii Fistulosi*	9 grams
蘆根	*Rhizoma Phragmatis Communis*	9 grams
甘草	*Radix Glycyrrhizae*	1.5 grams
神麯	*Massa Fermentata*	9 grams

If, after taking **Prescription III for Influenza**, above, and having sweated as directed, the patient still has some fever, coughing, or throat problems, then this prescription should be given. Boil the herbs in 3 cups of water until 1 cup remains and drink when warm.

The traditional Chinese pharmacist uses the *Ch'ien* (錢) (equal to approximately 3 grams) as the basic unit for weighing herbs in prescriptions.

Prescription V for Influenza		
Herb		Quantity
Chinese	Pharmaceutical Name	
藿香	*Herba Agastaches*	9 grams
白芷	*Radix Angelica Dahuricae*	6 grams
蘇梗	*Caulis Perillae*	9 grams
雲苓	*Sclerotium Polypori*	12 grams
陳皮	*Pericarpium Citri Reticulatae*	1.5 grams
桔梗	*Radix Platycodi Grandiflori*	7.5 grams
白术	*Rhizoma Atractylodis Macrocephalae*	6 grams
川星朴	*Rhizoma Ligustici*	9 grams
神麯	*Massa Fermentata*	9 grams
大腹皮	*Pericarpium Arecae*	9 grams
甘草	*Radix Glycyrrhizae*	3 grams
大棗	*Fructus Zizyphi Jujubae*	2 pieces
生薑	*Rhizoma Zingiberis Recens*	2 slices

Use this prescription in cases of flu accompanied by vomiting, diarrhea and/or abdominal pain. Most symptoms will disappear after one or two doses. Boil the herbs in 3 1/2 cups of water until only 1 cup remains and take when warm.

Prescription VI for Influenza		
Herb		Quantity
Chinese	Pharmaceutical Name	
• 柴胡	*Radix Bupleuri*	9 grams
• 半夏	*Rhizoma Pinelliae*	9 grams
• 黨參	*Radix Codonopsis*	9 grams
• 黃芩	*Rhizoma Coptidis*	9 grams
• 甘草	*Radix Glycyrrhizae*	3 grams
• 生薑	*Rhizoma Zingiberis*	2 slices
• 大棗	*Fructus Zizyphi Jujubae*	2 pieces
白眉	*Semen Vignae Cylindricae*	9 grams
白芍	*Radix Paeonia Lactiflora*	9 grams
小生地	*Radix Rehmanniae*	12 grams

This prescription may be used in cases of flu that has gone for several days without proper treatment, and which has entered the gallbladder meridian. The patient will have intermittent fever, a string pulse that is most evident on the left arm, a bitter taste in the mouth, and a thin white coating on the tongue. In this case, use the herbs preceded by "•" above, and boil in 3 cups of water until about 3/4 cup remains.

If a woman has a menstrual period during the flu, this situation is called *"the flu has entered the blood room [liver and heart]."* In this case, use all the herbs listed in the prescription, and boil in 3 1/2 cups of water until one cup remains. In both cases, wait until warm and then drink. One or two doses should bring about recovery.

The traditional Chinese pharmacist uses the *Ch'ien* (錢) (equal to approximately 3 grams) as the basic unit for weighing herbs in prescriptions.

Prescription VII for Influenza		
Herb		Quantity
Chinese	Pharmaceutical Name	
大黃	*Rhizoma Rhei*	9 grams
芒硝	*Magnesium Sulfate*	9 grams
枳實	*Fructus Ponciri*	9 grams
川朴	*Rhizoma Ligustici*	9 grams

This prescription may be used, *with caution*, in cases of flu that has gone for several days without proper treatment, and which has entered the large intestine meridian. The patient will have a high fever, a big and strong pulse, red and dry lips and tongue, a yellow coating on the tongue, constipation and possibly will be delirious *Do not use this prescription unless all the above symptoms are present.* After taking this prescription, the patient will move his or her bowels once or twice. This will be followed by recovery.

Boil herbs #1 and #2 in 2 cups of water for 2 minutes, then add herbs #3 and #4. Boil down to 3/4 of a cup, wait until warm, then let the patient drink it. One dose is all that is required.

The traditional Chinese pharmacist uses the *Ch'ien* (錢) (equal to approximately 3 grams) as the basic unit for weighing herbs in prescriptions.

Prescription VIII for Influenza		
Herb		Quantity
Chinese	Pharmaceutical Name	
石膏	*Calcium Sulfate*	60 grams
知母	*Rhizoma Anemarrhena*	9 grams
甘草	*Radix Glycyrrhizae*	3 grams
花粉	*Radix Tricosanthis*	9 grams
粳米	*Semen Oryzae*	30 grams

This prescription is for the flu which has been treated incorrectly and has changed into a high fever. The patient will be very thirsty, perspire copiously, and have a big and strong pulse. It is important to distinguish this case from the previous one. Note that this patient perspires; there is no perspiration in the previous case.

Boil the herbs in 3 cups of water until 1 cup remains and drink when warm.

Prescription IX for Influenza		
Herb		Quantity
Chinese	Pharmaceutical Name	
香薷	*Herba Elshotziae*	9 grams
扁豆	*Semen Lablab*	9 grams
川星朴	*Cortex Magnoliae Officinalis*	9 grams
甘草	*Radix Glycyrrhizae*	3 grams
川蓮	*Rhizoma Coptidis*	9 grams
雲苓	*Sclerotium Polypori*	12 grams
川木瓜	*Fructus Chaenomelis*	9 grams

This prescription is for sunstroke and a high fever, red face, thin white coating on tongue, and a floating pulse on both hands. These cases occur most frequently in southern climates, always in hot weather. Boil the herbs in 3 cups of water until 1 cup remains, and drink when warm.

Prescription X for Influenza		
Herb		Quantity
Chinese	Pharmaceutical Name	
甘草	*Radix Glycyrrhizae*	9 grams
桔梗	*Radix Platycodi*	9 grams
酒黃芩	*Radix Scutellariae*	9 grams
酒川蓮	*Rhizoma Coptidis*	9 grams
馬勃	*Fructificatio Lasiosphaerae*	3 grams
元參	*Radix Scrophulariae*	3 grams
橘紅	*Pericarpium Citri Erythrocarpae*	3 grams
柴胡	*Radix Bupleuri*	3 grams
羌蠶	*Bombyx cum Batryte*	3 grams
薄荷	*Herba Menthae*	3 grams
升麻	*Rhizoma Cimicifgae*	1.4 grams
連喬	*Fructus Forsythiae*	4.5 grams
牛蒡子	*Fructus Bardanae*	4.5 grams

This prescription is used specifically in cases of ''Frog Epidemic,'' which is characterized by high fever and swelling at the neck. Boil the herbs in 3 1/2 cups of water until 1 cup remains, and drink when warm. Three such doses may be required to effect a cure.

Prescription XI for Influenza		
Herb		Quantity
Chinese	Pharmaceutical Name	
香付	*Rhizoma Cyperi*	7.5 grams
甘草	*Radix Glycyrrhizae*	3 grams
陳皮	*Pericarpium Citri Reticulatae*	4.5 grams
蘇葉	*Folium Perillae*	7.5 grams
蓁艽	*Radix et Ramulus Malvae*	7.5 grams
京芥	*Herba Schizonepetae*	7.5 grams
川芎	*Rhizoma Ligustici*	6 grams
防風	*Herba Ledebouriellae*	6 grams
蔓荊子	*Fructus Viticis*	6 grams

This prescription is recommended at the beginning of a flu, when the pulse neither sinks nor floats. Boil the herbs in 3 cups of water until 1 cup remains, and drink when warm.

The traditional Chinese pharmacist uses the *Ch'ien* (錢) (equal to approximately 3 grams) as the basic unit for weighing herbs in prescriptions.

Cholera

Causes: This is an acute infection caused by *Vibrio cholerae*, cholera germs, entering the body through the mouth.

Symptoms: Before an attack, the germs may remain in the body for 1 to 8 days. In other cases, the cholera attack may come a few hours after infection. In the beginning, there will be mild diarrhea for 2 or 3 days, followed by the cholera attack itself.

During the cholera attack, the patient's body will become extremely weak, and, in 1 or 2 hours, will become thin. The diarrhea will be extremely frequent, often recurring more than 10 times in the space of one hour, accompanied by severe vomiting. Otherwise, there will be no other pain in the body.

In the beginning, the feces have a normal color, which, as the disease progresses, appears like watery milk, with small, milky-white pieces of fecal matter. There will be great thirst and borborygmus. The patient's face will be thin and emaciated, with the cheeks and eyeballs sinking in, and the cheek bones sticking out. The skin and mucus membrane are white and dry, and the mucus membranes may be cleft.

If the arms and legs are cold, the voice very feeble, with cramp in the calf of the legs and an imperceptible pulse, this indicates that the patient is dying.

The patient cannot pass urine because all the liquid in the body is absorbed into the intestines and leaves the body through the rectum or by vomiting. The patient suffers from palpitations of the heart and feels pressure on the heart. There is a great desire to sleep because of the growing weakness. The temperature under the armpit is below normal because the body is in a cold condition, but by taking the patient's temperature from the rectum it will be found to be very high.

In mild conditions, the attack may last 1 or 2 days, after which the patient will die; in severe conditions the patient will die in a few hours. If the condition alters and the vomiting ceases, the feces regain color and the patient is able to pass urine, he or she may recover in one or two weeks. However, with acupuncture treatment, even in very severe conditions, the patient will recover in one or two hours.

Treatment

• *Treatment of "Wet" Cholera (severe vomiting and diarrhea)*

Apply 1 direct moxa (yellow bean size or 1/2 peanut size) to CV-12, ST-25, CV-4, and CV-8 (use salt if the umbilicus is deep). For all points except CV-8, fix the moxa on the point with Vaseline, and burn all the moxa simultaneously. Have an assistant hold the patient so the he or she does not turn around during this procedure. This treatment will save the patient's life, and will cause the arms and legs to become warm, the pulse to return and the vomiting and diarrhea to cease. The patient should return to consciousness directly after this treatment. Additional applications of moxa may be used if necessary.

• *Treatment of "Dry" Cholera (inability to pass stool or vomit)*

Step One: Apply needle to GV-26.

Step Two: Apply triangular needle to LU-11, LI-1, PC-9, TW-1, HT-9, and SI-1. Draw out a few drops of blood form these points.

Step Three: Apply needle to LI-4, LI-11, and PC-5.

Step Four: Apply needle to GB-39, LV-3, ST-44, and BL-54. Draw out a few drops of blood from the vein near BL-54.

Step Five: Apply needle to CV-13, CV-12, and CV-10.

• *Treatment of Cholera with cramping of the feet and legs*

Treat as for "Wet Cholera", and apply 5 direct moxa (red bean size) to KI-1 and BL-57. If the cramp has not completely loosened, apply direct moxa on salt to CV-8 as many times as required to loosen the cramp.

• ***Treatment of cholera-like disorder,*** *sha* ***(twisted intestines)***

In this case, there is unrelieved pain in the entire abdomen, with cold hands, arms, legs and feet. Apply olive or peanut oil to the region 2-3 inches above and below LU-5, PC-3, and BL-54, rubbing a few drops of oil lightly into the skin with your fingers. Using a porcelain spoon, or a smooth-edged jar top, scratch downward on the skin on the oiled areas.

Apply oil on the back, from the shoulders to the lumbar region, and scratch in the same manner. Look for small red or dark spots that will appear on the surface of the skin as a result of this procedure. Pierce these with a triangular needle and draw out a few drops of blood. The pain will immediately cease, and recovery will be immediate. This oil and scratching may also be applied to the abdomen.

Should the above treatment be unsuccessful, bleed the fingertip well points.

Assistant Points (for cholera only): PC-3, BL-54 (draw out a few drops of blood from the vein close to this point), CV-13, LV-14, BL-21, TW-6, PC-5, GB-34, SP-9, SP-2, and KI-1.

Prognosis: One or two treatments.

Note: After treatment, give **Prescription V** for **Influenza**.

Inflammation

Causes: Inflammation of any part of the body is caused by some irritation of the skin. The severity of the irritation depends on the type of irritant and the reaction of the skin in the particular area of the irritation. Examples of irritants include chemicals, poisons, and, most commonly, germs.

Symptoms: Redness of the skin; swelling; pain; heat in the region of the irritation; hindrance of movement in the region.

Treatment

Step One: Apply needle to LI-11.

Step Two: Apply needle to SP-10 and BL-54.

Step Three: Apply needle to those points close to the region of the inflammation.

Step Four: Apply Rivenal (a German medicinal liquid) to the region of the inflammation.

Step Five: If there is pus in the inflamed region, or if there are signs of pus forming, and if the inflamed region is in the upper part of the body, apply 5 direct moxa (green bean size) to LI-11. If the inflamed region is in the lower part of the body, apply 5 direct moxa (green bean size) to SP-10. After moxa, apply Red Jade Ointment to the inflamed region. If both upper and lower parts of the body are inflamed with pus, apply direct moxa to LI-11 and SP-10, both on the same day, or LI-11 on the 1st day and SP-10 on the 2nd day. If the inflammation is chronic in nature, and if there has been an open sore for a long time, apply 7 direct moxa (red bean size) to BL-17, in addition to SP-10 and LI-11.

Step Six: If there is itch all over the body, apply needle to LI-11, SP-10, BL-54, and BL-13.

Prognosis: If the inflammation is no more than 2 to 3 days old, 1 or 2 treatments; if there is pus, 5 to 7 treatments. If long standing, up to 10 treatments will be required.

Furuncle, Blood Poisoning and Septicemia

In these conditions, a small pock mark appears, from which a red line emerges. If on the face, the red line progresses in the direction of the brain; if on the arm, it moves toward the arm pit; if on the foot or leg the red line will go up to the umbilicus. In all cases, the patient will develop a fever.

Causes: Streptococcic or staphylococcic germs enter through the hair follicles and cause inflammation and a small boil.

Symptoms: The small boil is hard and has a root in the flesh shaped like a nail. The Chinese call this a ''nail'' boil. The illness runs a very rapid course and the patient suffers from severe poisoning. Some patients suffering from such a condition may feel well in the morning and die within 10 to 12 hours; others die almost immediately. Still other cases may last a few days or as long as two weeks.

In the beginning, the boil has a tiny head and there is a little itchiness or, when scratched, numbness. Later, there is a little pain. In some cases, there is pain from the outset. If itch precedes the pain, the poison is much more severe, and is more likely to spread over the entire body. For 1 to 2 days the patient has a high fever and coldness in the body, especially in the back. In more serious conditions, the patient will vomit and will be very restless. The patient will feel dizzy and will not be able to see clearly. The tongue will not move freely and the mouth will be dry. The hands and legs will become cyanotic due to impaired circulation. The abdomen becomes swollen and the patient will be very weak and tired, often talking deliriously.

In some cases, the pimple or boil is very tiny; in other cases, it might be rounder, or longer, sometimes the size of a green bean, but never larger than a yellow bean. The color of the boil may be yellow, white, blue, or black. Some cases show no actual boil but only a red line. Septicemia is more common in the limbs than on the face or body.

If the red line which develops reaches the armpit (in cases of septicemia in the upper limbs), the umbilicus (in cases involving the lower limbs), or the throat (in cases of septicemia on the face, lips, or inside the mouth), the patient cannot be saved.

If the location of the septicemia is not apparent, and yet the patient suffers with high fever, a cold feeling, and all the symptoms listed above, after a few days there will be swelling in some part of the body, indicating that the septicemia is inside the body. In some patients, it may occur inside the armpit, the crotch, the scrotum, in the region of the anus or vagina, in the scalp covered by hair, or even under the nail. In all cases, the infected part must be located.

Special Diagnosis:

A) Give the patient several *raw* yellow beans to chew. If the patient says the taste of the yellow beans is pleasant and not at all offensive, this is a sign that the patient is suffering from septicemia.

B) If the dregs from the distillation of Chinese wine are placed in the patient's mouth and held for a few minutes before spitting them out, the patient will feel pain in the region of the septic focus.

C) If the patient vomits and the eyes are unable to move (the patient looks straight forward), or he or she is delirious, the patient cannot be cured.

Treatment

• *Treatment Method I*

Step One: Apply needle to GV-12 and GV-10.

Step Two: Apply needle to LI-4, LI-11, and PC-9. Draw out a few drops of blood with a triangular needle from PC-9.

Step Three: Apply needle to SP-10 and BL-54.

Step Four: Obtain a number of fresh wild chrysanthemum flowers and squeeze out 1 or 2 cups of juice from them. Have the patient drink the raw (uncooked) liquid. This will be found to be most helpful. If the fresh flower is unobtainable, go to the herbalist and buy one tael (1½ to 2 oz) of chrysanthemum, place it into 3 cups of water and boil down to 1 cup and give the patient to drink. This is not as effective as the fresh raw juice.

• ***Treatment Method II***

Apply 14 direct red bean size moxa to a point between the two tendons of the arm, 4 divisions distal from the base of the palm. One or two treatment will suffice.

• ***Treatment Method III***

In the early stages of septicemia, apply 7 direct moxa (red bean size) to PC-7 (with males, apply on the left arm; with females, on the right arm.) One treatment will suffice. In the last stages of septicemia, apply the triangular needle to the focus of the infection and squeeze out as much blood as possible. Follow the yellow line leading from the septic focus to its terminus. Here, the skin will be slightly raised and a small raised point on the skin, similar to a mosquito bite, may be found. Pierce this point with a triangular needle, pressing out as much blood as possible. At the terminus of the red line, apply 3 direct moxa (green bean size). If not already too late, this might save the patient's life.

• ***Treatment Method IV***

Septicemia occurring around the mouth is particularly dangerous (the Chinese call this "lock the mouth" septicemia). In this form of septicemia, the root will be found on the back, and will be visible as a small red point. If the septicemia is on the left corner of the mouth, the root will be found on the right side of the back. If the septicemia shows itself on the right side of the mouth, the root will be found on the left side of the back. In both instances, the root will be found above the waist.

Apply the triangular needle to the red point, piercing it and drawing out as much blood as possible. Next, take a few bitter almonds, place them in warm water and take off the skin. Pound the almonds and apply the pounded paste to the focus of the infection around the mouth. Change four times in 24 hours, using fresh pounded almonds in each instance.

• ***Treatment Method V***

For septicemia on the fingers, use the triangular needle to pierce the base line of the finger affected by the septicemia and draw out as much blood as possible. This will prevent the poison from going to the other fingers. If the poison has already spread to the other fingers, use the triangular needle to pierce the base line of all the affected fingers.

• *Treatment Method VI*

In the case of septicemia where there is a "nail" or "head" with a red line running from it, apply the triangular needle to the end of the red line, and squeeze out as much blood as possible. If the septicemia shows no "head" or "nail" but merely a red line, apply the triangular needle to both ends and the middle of the red line, and press out as much blood as possible.

• *Treatment Method VII*

Septicemia in the philtrum of the upper lip (on the Governing Vessel line) is very dangerous, and the poison is apt to spread very rapidly. Apply 10 direct moxa (red bean size) to LI-4 bilaterally.

Note: With each of *Treatment Methods II* through *VII*, *Treatment Method I* must also be used.

Prognosis: 2 to 5 treatments, depending to the seriousness of the case.

Prescription I for Septicemia
Apply the fresh blood of a cock's comb to the focus of the septicemia. This will be found to be a great help.

Prescription II for Septicemia
Apply the urine of a cat (preferably a male cat) on the region of the septic focus. (This is more potent than the first prescription.) To obtain the fresh urine of a cat, place the cat in a basin, get someone to hold down its legs, and rub the cat's nose with fresh ginger. Absorb some of the urine on cotton wool and apply this fresh urine on the "septic head."

Prescription III for Septicemia
Obtain 10 to 20 live bed bugs and put them into a bowl. Take half a table-spoon of hot boiled rice and place this rice into the same bowl. Grind the rice and live bed bugs together, so that the blood of the bed bugs is mixed with the rice paste. Apply the paste to the region of the septicemia. This is of no value where the septicemia has no "head" or "nail."

Carbuncles and Abscesses

Causes: An inflammatory condition of the skin and tissues under the skin, usually caused by staphylococcus entering through the root of the hair or the sweat glands. An immune system compromised by illness or general weakness allows the staph to grow unchecked. If the patient has suffered an injury to any part of the body, that region will be more susceptible to the carbuncle.

Symptoms: At first, the tissue under the skin feels hard and a little painful. The skin in the region turns red or even purple. As the swelling increases, so does the pain. Sometimes the swelling may have a diameter of a few inches. As the carbuncle enlarges, the center softens, and after a few days a few holes will be found in the center which exude pus and dead tissue. The hole enlarges day by day. If the dead tissue and pus are able to come out, new tissues will form and the carbuncle will heal. Carbuncles are most common on the back, neck, and arms, because in these parts there is less bodily movement. The fever accompanying a carbuncle may be quite high.

An abscess is not as severe as a carbuncle and not as dangerous. There is only one hole, and if the pus is allowed to drain, the patient can easily recover without difficulty.

Treatment

Step One: Apply needle to LI-11 and triangular needle to LU-11. Obtain a strong stimulus from the LU-11 and draw out a few drops of blood.

Step Two: Apply needle to SP-10, BL-54, and LV-1. Obtain a strong stimulus from LV-1.

Step Three: Apply needle to BL-17. If the patient has no fever, apply 7 direct moxa (red bean size) to BL-17. If there is a fever, do not apply direct moxa.

Step Four: Apply some Red Jade Ointment to the carbuncle. In the early stages, when there is still no pus in the carbuncle, after one or two treatments the patient will recover. If there is an open sore, wash it thoroughly with carbolic liquid, Chinese tea or some other strong disinfectant before applying the medicine referred to under **Prescriptions for Inflammations**. Usually 3 or 4 treatments will suffice in more advanced conditions. The same treatment is used for abscesses.

Note: If the condition worsens, and the carbuncle is in the upper part of the body, the sore is open, and the fever is reduced, apply 5 direct moxa (red bean size) to LI-11. If the carbuncle is in the lower part of the body, apply 5 direct moxa (red bean size) to SP-10 and apply White Ointment or Red Jade Ointment.

Prognosis: Three to five treatments are necessary. If the condition is very bad, it may require up to 7 treatments.

Cold Abscess

This is a chronic form of abscess caused by the tubercle bacillus. The patient is weak and pale. The abscess is not red, but is the same color as the skin of the body, with some swelling and a little pain. The condition is very chronic and may take months or even a year before it becomes an open sore. The abscess will be long or wide, like an underground passage under the skin. Once the sore opens, it is difficult to heal, and pus and foul liquid exude from it. The patient lingers on and gradually weakens and dies. Sometimes the cold abscess may open in some other part or parts of the body. In the beginning, the patient does not suffer much and is able to walk around, eat, work. However, after the sore opens, the patient loses strength and weakens rapidly.

Treatment

Apply the same acupuncture treatment as for **Carbuncle**, except that more direct moxa should be used. In addition, add the following steps:

On the first day: apply 7 direct moxa (red bean size) to LI-11.
On the second day: apply 7 direct moxa (red bean size) to SP-10.
On the third day: apply 7 direct moxa (red bean size) to BL-17.
On the fourth day: apply 7 direct moxa (red bean size) to BL-18.

Apply these steps whether or not the sore is open.

Though not absolutely necessary in the case of cold abscess, acupuncture will be a great help. Direct moxa treatment, however, is essential. Ten direct moxa can also be applied to BL-38 (red bean size) and 5 direct moxa (red bean size) to GV-4, as soon as the patient has nearly recovered or after recovery. The treatment using these two points will help the patient regain bodily strength.

Note: This condition is rare among North Americans and Europeans. When it does occur in these cultures, the moxa treatment mentioned above will, in most cases, be unacceptably intense. In Asia and South America, however, where this condition is most common, this treatment may be attempted without fear of offense.

Ringworm

Causes: This is caused by a fungus. It is easy to contract and spreads easily to other parts of the body.

Symptoms: Ringworm can develop on any area of the skin. Although it is generally round in shape, it may also appear elongated. It may focus in one small area of the body, appear as rings in several areas at once, or spread over a wide area of the skin. If the ringworm is in the nape of the neck, the back of the wrist, or the front of the ankle, it is more difficult to cure and may cause the skin to thicken considerably. When the skin thickens in this way, the Chinese call it "cow's skin ringworm." It is very difficult to cure. The skin will be very itchy in the region. In some early stages, even without treatment the patient may recover completely; in other cases, mild treatment will suffice. In other cases, no matter what treatment the patient is given, there will be no recovery. In still other cases, the ringworm will recover in some parts of the body only to break out afresh in another. In certain cases, the ringworm will occur symmetrically over the body.

Treatment

Step One: Apply needle to LI-11.

Step Two: Apply needle to BL-13 and BL-17.

Step Three: Apply needle to SP-10 and BL-54.

Step Four: Apply indirect moxa with instrument to the region of the ringworm. Initially during this procedure, the patient will feel more itchy, and as the moxa continues to heat the skin, the patient will feel some pain. To help alleviate this, apply finely crushed garlic to the region being treated.

In cases of ringworm in its early stages (though not when the ringworm has spread over the body), the above treatment applied 4 to 7 times will suffice.

Step Five: **For advanced cases and ''cow's skin'' ringworm**: First apply **Steps One** to **Three**, above. With a needle, prick gently all over the region of the ringworm, drawing a little blood from the skin pricks. Wipe away the blood after squeezing it out of the skin. Then apply indirect moxa with instrument. Continue with the indirect moxa instrument until the itch stops, and apply the crushed garlic all over the affected area. In some cases, the patient will respond rapidly.

Prognosis: In the early stages, 3 to 7 treatments will suffice. In advanced stages, particularly the ''cow's skin'' ringworm, it may take a few months to bring about a cure. As mentioned above, in some cases the disease cannot be cured.

Scabies

Causes: Scabies are caused by a tiny insect that burrows into the skin, causing pimples to erupt. The pimples will fill with liquid, and eventually dry up, leaving a dark spot at the site. This dark color consists of the feces of the insect. As the insect burrows deeper, another pimple will arise, where the scabies insect will breed. This process continues as the scabies spread over the whole body. Scabies may be transmitted from one person to another, and usually appear between the fingers, on the abdomen, penis or scrotum, the inguinal creases, the feet, or the buttock. Scabies never occur on the face. They more commonly occur in the warm weather.

Symptoms: Itch in the affected region, especially at night when the patient is covered up in bed. Sometimes scratching the itch causes the scabies pimples to erupt with pus.

Treatment

Step One: Apply needle to LI-11 and LI-5.

Step Two: Apply needle to BL-13 and BL-17.

Step Three: Apply needle to SP-10 and BL-54.

Step Four: If the patient has been suffering from scabies for a long time, or if there is pus in the scabies pimple, apply 5 direct moxa (red bean size) to LI-11 and SP-10.

Prognosis: Up to 7 treatments should suffice. Usually only application with the needle will suffice.

Chillblains

Causes: Chillblains occur in cold weather and are due to poor circulation of the blood at the extremities, particularly the toes, fingers, ears, and occasionally the nose. People suffering from anemia or malnourishment are more susceptible to chillblains.

Symptoms: Chillblains occur in three stages:

Stage One: The capillaries at the extremities become constricted and the skin appears very white. If the cold weather continues, the extremities feel numb. Due to poor circulation, the affected parts will swell and take on a purplish or blue color, with severe itch, particularly at night in bed.

Stage Two: The swollen parts will show liquid inside and then the skin breaks and a small ulcer may appear.

Stage Three: The condition becomes severe, and pus may exude from the ulcer which continues to enlarge. The color will deepen, and the blood will not circulate. If this condition is not remedied, even the bones may become destroyed.

Treatment

Apply indirect moxa with fresh ginger on the affected chillblains until the part is hot as the patient can bear. The treatment should be repeated 2 to 3 times each day until the itch has completely ceased. In 3 to 5 days, the patient should be well again.

For ulcerated chillblains, with pus and liquid, light a quantity of moxa (pigeon's egg size) on a saucer or other suitable container. While burning, allow the chillblains to rest over the fumes without touching the burning moxa. Alternately, use a moxa instrument to blow the burning fumes onto the affected parts. Repeat the treatment 2 or 3 times each day. The patient will be cured in 5 to 7 days.

Prognosis: In its first stage, chillblains may be treated in 1 or 2 treatments; in its last stage, 5 to 7 treatments will be required.

Corns and Warts

Treatment

Apply 5 to 7 direct moxa the size of the head of the corn, to the corn. One or two treatments will suffice. The root of the corn or wart will die and drop out in a few days.

For a corn or wart under the foot, it is necessary to apply several treatments using 10 yellow bean size moxa each time. After each treatment, the foot should be soaked in a basin of hot water and should remain in the water until the water has cooled down. After 3 to 5 treatments, the patient is usually cured. During the treatment, the patient should walk as little as possible.

Excessive Sweating or Night Sweating

Causes: Normal sweating or perspiring is due to physical work, heat, or sudden fright. Sweating may also be due to illness from physical weakness or from tuberculosis.

Symptoms:: Perspiration occurring in the daytime, in the absence of physical exertion, heat or sudden fright, and profuse perspiration that occurs during sleep are considered disorders. A related disorder is profuse sweating under the armpit accompanied by offensive odor.

Treatment

Step One: Apply needle to LI-4, HT-6, and SI-3.

Step Two: Apply needle to KI-7 and KI-8.

Step Three: In mild conditions, apply indirect moxa with ginger to HT-6 and KI-7. In severe conditions, add 3 direct moxa (green bean size) to these points.

If the patient is very weak after successful completion of the above treatment, he or she will likely suffer a recurrence of the condition. To prevent this, apply 5 direct moxa (red bean size) to BL-38 and 3 direct moxa (green bean size) to ST-36. Continue with the direct moxa treatment alone for 3 to 5 days. If there is excessive sweating in the hands, in addition to the above treatment apply 3 direct moxa (green bean size) to SI-3 and HT-6. This treatment should be given daily for three days. Should this not be successful, apply 5 direct moxa (red bean size) to BL-15. If the excessive sweating is in the feet, in addition to the above treatment, apply needle to BL-54, and 5 direct moxa (green bean size) to KI-2. If there is offensive odor under the armpits from sweating, apply 5 direct moxa (green bean size) to HT-1.

Prescription for Children's Night Sweating	
Step One	Grind an ounce of *Wu Bui Tzy* into powder.
Step Two	Take a quantity of this powder sufficient to fill the hole in the umbilicus of the child, and with a little spittle of the child (if a baby, with a little of the mother's spittle) or even with a little water, mix the powder into a sticky paste.
Step Three	Apply the paste to the umbilicus of the child just before the child goes to bed at night. Remove it in the morning. Apply 3 to 4 such treatments. Acupuncture will not be necessary.

Prescription for Offensive Odor Under the Arms	
Step One	Grind 1 oz. of *Jeung Noh,* 1 oz. of *Mut Tar junk,* and 1/5 oz. of *Heng Fun* together.
Step Two	Mix 2 tsp. of the powder with 1 tsp. vinegar to form a paste.
Step Three	Apply this paste to the armpits before retiring at night, and wash it off in the morning.
Step Four	Continue this treatment for three nights in succession. Thereafter, apply once each week. It should be noted that this is not a cure, but rather will help reduce the odor while acupuncture treatment is being performed.

Prescription I for Sweating		
Herb		Quantity
Chinese	Pharmaceutical Name	
北芪	*Radix Huangchi*	15 grams
浮小麥	*Semen Marcidum Tritici*	9 grams
牡蠣	*Concha Ostreae*	9 grams
炙甘草	*Radix Glycyrrhizae*	3 grams
大棗	*Fructus Zizyphi Jujubae*	3 pieces

The above prescription may be used for excessive sweating and/or night sweating. Use 3 cups water, boil down to less than 1 cup, drink when warm. One should take 7 to 10 such doses.

Prescription II for Sweating		
Herb		Quantity
Chinese	Pharmaceutical Name	
樟腦	*Camphora*	6 grams
枯凡	*Lythargyrum*	3 grams
輕粉	*Calomelas*	6 grams
密陀僧	*Alumen*	3 grams

The above prescription may be used in cases of offensive odor under the armpits. Mix the above herbs and grind into a fine powder. Mix with a little vinegar to form a paste, and apply this mixture to the armpit before going to sleep. Apply every night for one week. After one week, apply once each week; the offensive odor will be gone.

The traditional Chinese pharmacist uses the *Ch'ien* (錢) (equal to approximately 3 grams) as the basic unit for weighing herbs in prescriptions.

Prescriptions for Digestive Disorders

Prescription I for Digestive Disorders		
Herb		Quantity
Chinese	Pharmaceutical Name	
黨參	*Radix Codonopsis*	9 grams
白術	*Rhizoma Atractylodes Macrocephalae*	9 grams
雲苓	*Lingchi*	12 grams
炙甘草	*Radix Glycyrrhizae*	3 grams
陳皮	*Pericarpium Citri Reticulatae*	6 grams
半夏	*Rhizoma Pinelliae*	9 grams
木香	*Radix Muhsiang*	9 grams
砂仁	*Semen et Pericarpium Amomi*	6 grams

In cases of poor digestion or lack of chi in the body, use herbs 1-4 only. If the patient also shows signs of overcooling and/or has a lot of phlegm, use herbs 1-7; when this condition is accompanied by gas in the abdomen, add herb #8. Boil the herbs in 3 cups of water (if only 4 herbs are used) or 3 1/2 cups of water (when 8 herbs are used), until one cup remains.

Prescription II for Digestive Disorders		
Herb		Quantity
Chinese	Pharmaceutical Name	
川芎	*Rhizoma Ligustici*	9 grams
當歸	*Angelica Sinensis*	9 grams
熟地	*Radix Rehmanniae Preparata*	12 grams
白芍	*Radix Paeonia Lactiflora*	9 grams
黃芪	*Radix Astragali*	9 grams
玉桂	*Cortex Cinnamomi*	3 grams

In cases of blood deficiency and poor circulation, use herbs 1-4 only. When there is insufficient chi and blood, add to herbs 1-4 of this prescription, herbs 1-4 of **Prescription I**, above. If the body is extremely weak and overcooling, combine all the herbs of this prescription with herbs 1-4 of **Prescription I**; this is called the ''Ten Tonifications.'' Boil the herbs in 3 cups of water (when 4 herbs are used) or 4 cups of water (if 8 to 10 herbs are used) until one cup remains.

Note: Overheating patients, or those with strong bodies, should not take this prescription.

Prescription III for Digestive Disorders		
Herb		Quantity
Chinese	Pharmaceutical Name	
白術	*Rhizoma Atractylodes Macrocephalae*	9 grams
北芪	*Radix Astragali Mongholicus (Pei-Ch'i)*	9 grams
茯神	*Poria Cocus (Fushen)*	9 grams
黨參	*Radix Codonopsis*	9 grams
遠志	*Radix Polygalae*	9 grams
木香	*Radix Muhsiang*	9 grams
棗仁	*Semen Ziziphi Spinosae*	9 grams
炙甘草	*Radix Glycyrrhizae*	3 grams
龍眼肉	*Arillis Longanae*	6 grams
當歸	*Radix Angelica Sinensis*	9 grams

The above prescription is effective in cases of weakness of the spleen, with pale face and lips, and tired muscles of the whole body. Boil the herbs in 3 1/2 cups of water until one cup remains.

Prescription IV for Digestive Disorders		
Herb		Quantity
Chinese	Pharmaceutical Name	
白術	*Rhizoma Atractylodes Macrocephalae*	9 grams
澤瀉	*Rhizoma Alismatis*	9 grams
茱苓	*Sclerotium Polypori*	9 grams
雲苓	*Sclerotium Poriae*	9 grams
玉桂心	*Cortex Cinnamomi*	1/3 grams

In cases of overcooling diarrhea and *supp,* use the entire prescription; for overheating of the bladder resulting in difficult urination (dysuria), use only herbs 1-4. Boil the herbs in 3 cups of water until 1 cup remains.

Prescription V for Digestive Disorders		
Herb		Quantity
Chinese	Pharmaceutical Name	
葛根	*Radix Puerariae*	12 grams
川蓮	*Rhizoma Ligustici*	9 grams
黃芩	*Radix Astragali vel Huangchi*	9 grams
生甘草	*Radix Glycyrrhizae*	9 grams

The above prescription is effective in cases of overheating diarrhea that are difficult to cure, with the accompanying symptom of a burning sensation in the anus. Boil the herbs in 2 1/2 cups of water until less than 1 cup remains.

Prescription VI for Digestive Disorders		
Herb		Quantity
Chinese	Pharmaceutical Name	
雲苓	*Sclerotium Poriae*	15 grams
土茯苓	*Sclerotium Polypori*	15 grams
沒藥	*Myrrha*	4.5 grams
冬瓜仁	*Semen Benincasae*	15 grams
敗醬草	*Herba Sonchi Brachyot*	9 grams

The above prescription is effective in cases of inflammation of the caecum or appendicitis in the first stage. Boil the herbs in 3 cups of water until 1 cup remains. Take once a day, for several days.

The traditional Chinese pharmacist uses the *Ch'ien* (錢) (equal to approximately 3 grams) as the basic unit for weighing herbs in prescriptions.

Prescription VII for Digestive Disorders		
Herb		Quantity
Chinese	Pharmaceutical Name	
川萆薢	*Rhizoma Smilacis*	9 grams
黃柏	*Cortex Phellodendri*	6 grams
石菖蒲	*Herba Acori Graminei*	3 grams
雲苓	*Sclerotium Poriae*	9 grams
白術	*Rhizoma Atractylodes Macrocephalae*	6 grams
蓮心	*Embryon Nelumbinis*	6 grams
丹參	*Radix Salviae Miltiorhizae*	6 grams
車前子	*Semen Plantaginis*	6 grams

The above prescription is effective in cases of urethral discharge or for the beginning stages of gonorrhea. Boil the herbs in 3 cups of water, until one cup remains.

Prescription VIII for Digestive Disorders		
Herb		Quantity
Chinese	Pharmaceutical Name	
木棉花	*Radix et Flos Bombacis*	9 grams
川萆薢	*Rhizoma Peihsieh (Szechuan)*	9 grams
炒扁豆	*Semen Dolichoris*	9 grams
赤小豆	*Semen Phaseoli Calcarati*	9 grams
薏仁	*Semen Coicis*	9 grams
土茯苓	*Sclerotium Poriae*	15 grams

The above prescription may be used effectively for overheating and *supp,* which may be indicated by such symptoms as deep yellow urine, soft and sticky bowel movement, and wet coating on the tongue. Boil the herbs in 3 cups of water until one cup remains. Add salt or sugar to taste.

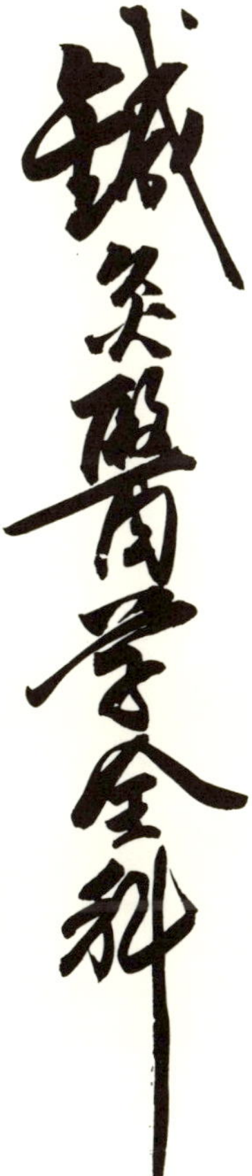

V

Case Reports

Case Reports

• *Case I: Leukemia*

Hong Kong, September 10, 1959

Mr. Mung Wing Cheong, 57, a merchant trading with Japan, was diagnosed as having leukemia. When the doctor at the hospital announced that Mr. Mung's life was to end within a few months, Mr. Mung went home to await his death.

Mr. Mung wrote a letter to a Japanese doctor and asked for help. The Japanese doctor recommended moxibustion, and soon Mr. Mung arrived at my clinic asking for treatment.

Mr. Mung's pulses revealed weak kidneys and heart, so I applied five direct moxa on BL-15 and GV-11. This treatment was repeated for two days, after which the patient felt renewed strength. This treatment was followed by the application of five direct moxa to GV-4 and BL-23, again for two days. Mr. Mung's energy and strength were restored. As a third step, five direct moxa were applied to BL-20. In addition, at least three moxa were applied to LI-10 and ST-36 to increase his appetite.

Mr. Mung is healthy and strong to this day, and has put on some weight.

• *Case II: Leukemia*

Kuala Lumpur, Malaysia, 1965

In 1965, I visited Malaysia and met my friend Mr. Yip. Mr. Yip's 60 year old friend Mr. Chan Chuck Fu had leukemia. Mr. Chan was being treated at a church hospital, and his condition was becoming life-threatening. His eyes were dim, and the people whom he saw appeared headless. He could not distinguish colors, and there was blood in his urine. His abdomen had a number of spots.

Mr. Yip asked if I could use moxibustion to cure Mr. Chan. I told him that although I had been able to help a similar case, this patient's condition was considerably worse, and, moreover, this patient was elderly and the disease was at its height. However, I assured him that I would do my best.

I first applied five direct moxa on GV-4, each red-bean size. When I returned to see Mr. Chan the next day, there was no more blood in his urine. Five direct moxa were then applied to BL-23. On the third day, the patient's eyes were no longer dim, and he could distinguish colors, and recognize those who came to visit him. He could also speak distinctly.

On the fourth day, five moxa were applied to GV-11 and BL-15. Now he could wash his face and hands by himself, and help feed himself. The spots on his abdomen had also disappeared.

So that he could be thoroughly examined and a blood transfusion given, a hospital visit had been scheduled for the fifth day. Although the attending physician noticed the moxa scars and realized that a traditional Chinese doctor had been treating this patient, he believed that leukemia was incurable, and dismissed the moxibustion intervention as superfluous. Following the blood transfusion, Mr. Chan's pulse became more full, his blood no longer deteriorated, and he felt generally much better.

Finally, I applied moxa to BL-20. Having had every reason to believe that I had succeeded in helping Mr. Chan, I left Kuala Lumpur for Ipoh, another Malasian city. Soon, however, I heard that Mr. Chan caught pneumonia from the patient in the next hospital bed, and died within two days. Mr. Yip wrote to me to say that his friend had died not from blood cancer, but from pneumonia. It was a great pity.

Commentary: These first two case reports are factual, reported not for my own sake but to help acupuncturists in every country treat this disease.

The principles of Chinese therapeutics may be used to explain the efficacy of moxibustion in these cases. As you know, the bone marrow is the sight for the reproduction of red corpuscles. A patient having more white corpuscles would have less red ones because of the abnormality of the bone marrow. Since, according to traditional Chinese medical theory, the kidneys are the masters of the bone and bone marrow, and since the red corpuscles cannot be synthesized because of overcooling in the marrow, we may conclude that there exists a condition of overcooling in the kidney as well. Overcooling refers to a lowered body temperature, which decreases its capacity for synthesis.

Moxibustion on GV-4 and BL-23 can strengthen the kidneys and thus the marrow, thereby restoring the body's normal red corpuscle production.

The normal action of regulation and secretion of urine by the kidneys is also adjusted, thus clearing the condition of hematuria.

Again according to traditional Chinese medical theory, the blood and pulses are controlled by the heart. If the heart is weak, the blood's function would also be abnormal. Moxibustion on GV-11 and BL-15 was performed to strengthen the heart, further supporting the production of healthy red blood corpuscles.

The large increase in white corpuscles is due, in part, to the functioning of the spleen, which, according to Chinese medicine, controls the blood volume. BL-20 was thus treated with moxa to return the spleen to its normal function, and to decrease the number of white blood corpuscles.

• *Case III: Treatment of Headache with GV-4*

Kowloon, Hong Kong, Autumn, 1940

A 40 year old ship watchman had a headache as a result of catching the flu. After recovering from the flu, the headache persisted as he continued to work from midnight to eight in the morning as the ship's watchman. When this man came to my graduate student, Leung Mo Chih, for treatment, he had had these headaches for two years.

In the beginning, my student treated the patient with LI-4, LU-7, GB-20, GV-16, ST-8, GV-20, GV-24 and GV-4. Indirect moxa was used on GV-20 and GV-24. Following this treatment, the headache disappeared, only to return again the next morning after a full night's work on the ship. This pattern of treatment, relief of symptoms, and return of the headaches after work continued for three days. Finally, my student came to me for advice.

Understanding this type of condition, I advised my student to burn 5 red-bean size moxa on GV-4 after his normal treatment. After this treatment, the headaches never returned.

Commentary: This patient's headache was related to his work schedule. According to Chinese medicine, working at night causes "empty fire." Night work caused the body's energy or "fire" to go to the top of the head, so that the headache could not be relieved. Application of moxa to GV-4 caused this fire to sink, and thus to relieve the headaches. In cases of high blood pressure or in strong bodies, use a needle rather than moxa on this point for similar cases.

• *Case IV: Constipation in Infants*

Christian Chapel of Assembly Church, Shih Doh District, Kwang Si Province, Mainland China, Spring, 1943

The patient, the 15 day-old son of the preacher of the church, had been constipated for the past 7 days. Though not an unusual problem, constipation in such a young child is quite unnatural. Since Shih Doh District is quite small, there were no hospitals, drug stores or mineral oil available. Chinese herbs, which were available, are too strong for such young infants. The father of this baby therefore asked me if acupuncture might be useful. I said it would.

First, I used a needle on CV-6, inserting it to a depth of 1/8 inch and manipulating it for 5 seconds. Next, I inserted a needle at GV-1 to a depth of 1/4 inch, manipulating it for ten seconds. I treated the baby before noon, and by three o'clock that same afternoon, the baby had a bowel movement. The baby had a second bowel movement at 9 PM and a third at midnight. The baby was normal after that.

Commentary: The name of the point CV-6 is *Sea of Chi* and helps move all the Chi of the body. GV-1 stimulates the rectum.

A possible cause of this ailment is the mother's consumption of rich or overheating food during pregnancy or while nursing, causing a condition of overheating in the baby.

• *Case V: Moxibustion in the Treatment of Severe Diarrhea*

Hong Kong, 1942, approximately three weeks after the Japanese occupation of Hong Kong

Perhaps as a result of the deteriorated living conditions and lack of available good food in Hong Kong during the occupation, this middle aged man, a friend of Chang Boh San, one of my students, had been having diarrhea 30 times each day. He tried every medication as well as Chinese herbs, to no avail. He was growing weak, pale, and his condition was becoming dangerous.

Upon visiting his friend one evening, Chang Boh San noticed that something was quite wrong. Upon inquiring, he was told of his friend's problem, and his fear of dying because of his steadily deteriorating condition. Mr. Chang told him not to be afraid, that he was an acupuncture student, and would treat him immediately.

Chang Boh San applied moxa to GV-1. Although his friend experienced a great deal of pain, he endured it in the hope that this treatment would save his life. After 15 soybean size moxa, the patient felt much stronger, and much different. Mr. Chang applied ten more moxa to insure an adequate effect. As a result of these 25 moxa, the patient was able to sit up, talk, and laugh as though he had never been sick.

Commentary: This case was critical, and the patient may not have survived without such treatment. Thus it is that the points on the body are like the keys to a safe.

• *Case VI: Tuberculosis in the Vertebra*

Spring, 1945

A 35 year old farmer came to me for treatment after not being able to walk with a straight back for two years. There was pain, inflammation and swelling (but no reddening of the skin) at the seventh thoracic vertebra, which was hot to the touch. If the skin had been red, and the duration of the illness less than two years, the diagnosis would probably have been carbuncles or abscess (neither carbuncles nor abscesses last as long as two years). The probable cause of the ailment was penetration of tuberculosis germs into the vertebrae.

In the beginning of treatment, I needled BL-54, GV-10, and GV-9, and applied indirect moxa with ginger on the swollen bone. The pain was relieved. On the next treatment, I used the same points, with seven direct moxa on GV-10 and GV-9, the points directly above the seventh thoracic vertebra. Following this treatment, both the swelling and the pain were much relieved.

On the third treatment, I applied 7 direct red bean size moxa to both sides of the seventh thoracic vertebra, on the edge of the bone. On the fourth day, almost all the swelling was gone.

On the last treatment, I applied 5 moxa to the top of the bone. The patient had no pain by this time, and could walk with a straight back. Two months after teatment, the patient was as strong as he had been before the illness, and could carry 100 lbs. of food on his back to the country market to sell.

Commentary: Germs can only be killed by the application of direct moxa. In this case, the germs had lodged in the vertebrae, and thus it was necessary to burn moxa around the entire bone to destroy them.

• *Case VII: Treatment of the Chest Following Injury by a Gun Handle*

Shih Doh District, Kwang Si Province, Mainland China, Autumn, 1942

I grew up in Hong Kong, where only those with special permits could carry guns. Therefore, I never went hunting in Hong Kong, and never learned to handle a gun.

Following the Japanese occupation, I left Hong Kong in 1942 and moved to Kwang Si Province, where I treated patients each morning. One day, a neighbor asked me to go hunting with him after I finished seeing my patients. This friend loaned me a gun for the expedition, thinking that I knew how to use it. I thought that I would be able to handle it and didn't ask him for any instruction.

At a forest about a mile from town, we saw a big bird in a tree. I was to shoot first. I held the gun up, pulled the trigger, and was hit on the chest, at ST-18, by the recoiling rifle. The pain was intense, and I was left speechless and nearly fainted. Not being able to hunt the bird, I hunted myself! Throwing the gun to the ground, I turned and walked slowly home. I couldn't even respond to my friend's concerned questions.

The area around ST-18, where I had been hit by the handle, was red and swollen. After lying on my bed to determine a course of action, and knowing that there was no other doctor in town, nor anyone else who could help me, I decided to treat myself.

I placed moxa the size of a fingertip on the painful spot and burned them. After three such moxa, I was much more comfortable. Deep breathing was no longer painful. After two more moxa, the pain was entirely gone, and, to the great surprise of my neighbor, I was soon able to stand, walk and talk without hindrance.

Thirty years have passed since that episode, and I have never had any problem as a result of it.

Commentary: The rapid cure in this case was due to the fact that the problem was treated almost immediately, and to the large size of the moxa used. Moxa has the ability to relieve nerve pain, to increase local circulation, and to get rid of stagnant blood.

• *Case VIII: Injury from Bee Stings*

Shin Doh District, Kwang Si Province, Mainland China, Summer, 1943

The 35 year old farmer mentioned in the treatment for tuberculosis of the vertebra had a big tree in his front yard, which held a large hive of bumble bees (called "tiger bees" in China). Afraid that his children would get stung by the bees while playing outside, he decided to move the nest.

Wearing only shorts, and taking with him a long bamboo pole, he climbed up the tree to accomplish his task. What our friend had in the way of courage, he lacked in wisdom. No sooner had he struck the nest, than the bees swarmed and attacked him, stinging his face, neck, chest, and legs while he was still perched in the tree. Jumping down, he plunged himself into a pool of water, covered himself with clay, and ran to my house for help.

When he arrived at my house, his body was covered with several hundred bee stings, and he felt as though he were burning up. I immediately cleaned his body with water, then needled LI-4, LI-11, SP-10, BL-54 and GB-20. The burning lessened, and he was able to sit comfortably. At this time, I had been living in a Christian Chapel. The missionary before me left a large bottle of ammonia, which I opened and rubbed on the stings. This made the patient feel much better. When the ammonia dried, I applied mercurochrome to all the stings. In three days, he recovered.

Commentary: Any insect bite will cause inflammation. Therefore I used LI-11, SP-10, and BL-54, the major inflammation points. GB-20 was used to relieve his head pain. Ammonia (a base) was used to neutralize the acid of the venom. Mercurochrome was used to reduce the inflammation.

• *Case IX: Treatment of Burns*

Chong Ng District, Kwang Si Province, Winter, 1942

Winters in Kwang Si Province are very cold. To keep warm, people burn fires in basins about a foot high. A four year old child, standing near the fire, was accidentally pushed by his playmates so that he sat on the fire, burning his buttocks quite severely.

I happened to be in the next room, and came in at the call of the child's mother. I first needled LI-11, SP-10, BL-54 and GB-30 to decrease the pain and the inflammation. Next I used cotton wool soaked in alcohol, which I rubbed on the child's buttocks. The alcohol cooled the child's skin, stopped the pain and inflammation, and the child ceased crying. When the first piece of cotton became warm, another was placed on the skin. This was repeated three times. By sunset, the child felt comfortable, and was able to sleep. The following day, the child's buttocks were fine.

Commentary: In the old Chinese prescription books, ginger juice mixed with white wine is recommended for the treatment of burns. Rubbing alcohol was not available in those times; however, we know that white wine is 30% alcohol. One day I burnt my finger on a match. After dipping the burnt finger in a bowl of rubbing alcohol, I noticed that there was a great deal of relief. When the bowl of alcohol got warm, I replaced it with another. From this, I decided that alcohol was better than the ancient mixture of ginger and white wine for burns. I have used alcohol in burn treatments successfully over one hundred times. The concentration of the alcohol used in such cases should be 75%.

• *Case X: Miscarriages*

Kowloon, Hong Kong, Summer, 1952

A 25 year old woman, the wife of a sailor, had been quarreling with a woman at work. The following day, she began to hemorrhage. Not knowing that she was pregnant (this was a very young and ignorant couple), her husband came to ask for my help. Neither wanted her to go to the hospital. When I palpated this young woman's abdomen, I felt something resembling a large, hard ball moving inside. After questioning her more closely, I determined that she was at least five months pregnant, and that she was having a miscarriage.

Since she had been bleeding for eight days, I knew that it would be difficult to save the baby. I therefore helped the baby come out. First, I needled LI-4, SP-6, BL-60, ST-25, CV-4, BL-67, and Tok Yum. Then, I applied five moxa to Tu Yin, three moxa to BL-67, and five moxa to CV-4, all green bean size. The baby came out after 15 minutes.

After resting for a few days, the woman was able to return to work. After several months, she became pregnant again, and was able to carry her baby to full term. In this case, because the hemorrhaging had lasted so long, I felt that there was no way to save the baby. The probable cause of this miscarriage was malnourishment, excessive work and quarreling, which made the women's mind upset and uneasy.

• *Case XI: High Fever*

My Friend's House, Hong Kong, March 15, 1954

The ten year-old son of my friend, Mr. Pong, had had a fever of 104.8 °F for two days, his pulse rate was as high as 138 and he was delirious. The medical doctor's injections were of no benefit, and the Chinese herbs that had been prescribed only brought the fever down to 104 °F. Although Mr. Pong did not believe in acupuncture, he finally asked my help, which I gave on the condition that I be allowed to treat in the manner that I knew best.

At first I bled the twelve Well points on the boy's fingers with a prismatic needle. The darkest blood came from LI-1 and TW-1. Next, I needled LI-4, LI-11, BL-54, and KI-1, moving the needle for 30 seconds on KI-1.

After this treatment the boy perspired profusely and then regained consciousness, asking for water. Finally, he fell asleep. The next day, he was able to play in the family living room. Now, he has children of his own.

• *Case XII: Hemiplegia Cured by Electric Machine*

Kowloon, Hong Kong, December, 1958

Mr. Au, a 46 year old merchant, enjoyed drinking wine and sleeping late, a habit that often results in high blood pressure. One day, he woke up to find the left side of his body and face paralyzed. He was not able to talk clearly, and was drooling. Five days later, his wife, an ex-Sunday school friend of mine, told me that her husband had had a stroke, and asked for my help.

Upon arriving at Mr. Au's house, I took his pulse, which was slow, sinking, and soft, with a rate was 45-50 beats per minute. These pulse signs indicated that Mr. Au's condition was not one of overheating, an important consideration in cases such as this.

First, I applied three direct moxa on GV-20 to help disperse the congested blood in the brain. Then I needled GV-26, SI-19, and ST-4, to treat the facial paralysis, and followed this with indirect moxa to all points. To help the arm paralysis, I needled LI-15, LI-11, and LI-4. For the leg, BL-54, GB-30, GB-34, GB-39, and BL-60 were needled. Indirect moxa with moxa instrument was then applied to all the points of the arm and leg.

Generally, direct moxa is recommended in these cases. However, because this patient was afraid of the pain, I changed my normal technique by applying electrical stimulation to all points with an electric machine. Electricity was applied for five minutes at a time, as strong as the patient could withstand. Electrical stimulation on the arm was followed by indirect moxa, then the leg was treated similarly.

With daily treatments, the patient was able to move the paralyzed arm and leg; after five days of such treatment, he could walk around the house. After ten days, he could go to the bathroom by himself, and after sixteen treatments, he was completely recovered. As of this writing, he remains healthy.

Commentary: The patient who receives acupuncture early after a stroke (within three months) will recover quickly. After six months, treatment becomes much more difficult. Patients between 40 and 50 years of age recover much more readily than patients over 50. If the stroke starts by the patient falling on the floor, treatment will be much more difficult, and more dangerous for the patient. If the stroke occurs while the patient is asleep, it will be easier to treat and not as dangerous. Cases with high blood pressure after the stroke are more difficult to cure than cases with low blood pressure.

• *Case XIII: Trachoma*

Hong Kong, Summer, 1947

Madame Jiu, a 40 year-old herb doctor, was inexperienced in the treatment of eye diseases. So when she herself was afflicted with small white spots the size of sesame seed tips on both upper and lower eyelids, with irritation and congestion of the sclera, she came to see me. Neither the hospital nor the eye specialist were able to help her.

After needling LI-4, LI-11, ST-8, BL-1, BL-2, BL-18, BL-20, BL-21, TW-23, and GB-1, and applying 7 1/3 rice grain size moxa on Dai Guu Kung, the tearing and pain decreased. After five daily treatments, the whiteheads decreased in number. After seven treatments, each subsequent treatment made more and more whiteheads disappear. After two weeks, the patient was completely recovered.

Commentary: According to Madame Jiu's medical doctor, this case of trachoma was due to an infection. According to Chinese medical theory, cases such as this are due to disorders of the spleen (the upper eyelid belongs to the spleen) and stomach (the lower eyelid belongs to the stomach), a long history of overheating, and *Supp.*

Trachoma is difficult to treat with medicine. Medical doctors can only use ointments to rub away the spots. Even Chinese herbalists have difficulty with this disease, and most acupuncture treatment books do not discuss its treatment. The treatment described above may also be used effectively for cases of catarrh and eye inflammation.

It is interesting to note the use of the additional points BL-20 and BL-21 in this treatment. These points are the Yu points of the spleen and stomach, respectively. I learned this theory from my herb teacher, and attribute the effectiveness of the treatment to it.

I have taught this case to many of my students, and several have found success with this treatment.

• *Case XIV: Whithering of the Face in a Young Man*

Hong Kong, 1947

In order to enhance the beauty of his face, 16 year old Mr. Lee had been washing for a number of years with a rough soap. However, the extreme alkaline properties of the soap caused the facial skin to lose its muscle tone, resulting in excessive wrinkling. For all Mr. Lee's cosmetic efforts, now, at 24, he had the complexion of an old man. Many medical experts, including dermatologists, were unable to help him.

I determined that a possible cause of this case could have been a weakening of the trigeminal nerve. Thus, I surmised, if the trigeminal nerve could be strengthened, perhaps the condition could be alleviated. Therefore, I used LI-4 and LI-11 for their control over the face; ST-8, GV-23, BL-2, TW-23, and direct moxa on GV-24 to strengthen the branch of the trigeminal nerve that controls the forehead; TW-21, SI-19, LI-20, and GV-26 to strengthen the branch of the trigeminal nerve that controls the upper cheek; and finally ST-6, ST-4, and CV-24 to strengthen the lower branch of the trigeminal nerve. After needing these points, I used indirect moxa on ginger on TW-21, SI-19, ST-6, ST-4, and CV-24 so that all the nerves of the face received heat stimulation.

After three days, the face started to improve. After three weeks, all the wrinkles disappeared and the skin was as smooth as a young man's face should be.

• *Case XV: Acute Blindness*

Hong Kong, Summer, 1956

The daughter of Mr. Lee, the secretary of the Hong Kong Herbal Association, had a terrible temper, and was easily angered. In addition, she liked to read novels, and would often read until late in the evening before falling asleep. Even though her right eye had been blind for many years, she would read every night with her one good eye.

One day Miss Lee woke up to find that she was blind in both eyes, and called her father in her fright to tell him of her condition. Mr. Lee took his daughter to many good doctors, but her condition did not improve. Ten days later, he brought her to me.

At first, I used the points recommended for general eye diseases: LI-4, ST-8, GB-15, BL-1, BL-2, TW-23, and GB-1. The next day, when she returned, there was no improvement. I was left with no choice but to advise her about her living habits. I had found from her pulse that her liver was too strong and her kidney too weak. This caused a deficiency of fire in the Life Door.

Although I had never treated such a case before, and though none of my acupuncture books presented any approach to the case, I remembered from my studies that GV-4 and BL-18 should be used to treat blindness. I treated BL-18 first, bilaterally, stimulating it for 30 seconds. This drew down the overheating of the liver. Next I needled, then applied 10 red bean sized direct moxa to GV-4. After this treatment, I had her father take her home.

The next day both father and daughter returned. Happily, the daughter said: "When I woke up this morning, I could see everything!" I treated her once more in the same way, except that I only used 5 direct moxa on GV-4.

When I later saw Mr. Lee on the street, he reported that his daughter had experienced no recurrence of her problem.

• *Case XVI: A Cure for Madness in a Single Treatment*

Basil Church, Dan Nan City, North Borneo, April, 1963

For several years, the 52 year-old woman who lived next to the church would talk nonsense all day long, and remain awake all night, singing. She refused to consult a doctor, and when she was taken to see one by her daughter and son-in-law, she would refuse to take the medication prescribed.

While I was staying in Dan Nan City for four days, her son-in-law convinced her to see me, which she did one evening at about eight o'clock. She wore an old-fashioned elegant dress, and many chains and necklaces around her neck, and carried a long-handled parasol. I could see immediately that her singing was due to a spleen disorder. Using a heater, I checked SP-1 bilaterally to determine the nature of the imbalance. I found that the left side felt the heat after 20 seconds, while the right side felt the heat after 60 seconds, showing that the right side was the weak one.

After needling HT-7 and PC-6 to strengthen her heart, and GB-20 and GV-16 to calm her mind, I treated the left BL-20 with a needle, and the right side BL-20 with three direct moxa.

From that treatment on, she was cured of her nightly singing, and was able to sleep the whole night through.

• *Case XVII: Coldness*

Hong Kong, Summer, 1946

During the Japanese occupation of Hong Kong, there were great shortages in good quality food, water, and medicine. As a consequence, the population suffered many more illnesses than was common. It was during this time that Mr. Leung, a 50 year old boss of a furniture company, came down with a flu. Following this, Mr. Leung's body was cold all the time, even during the summer. When I came to see him, Mr. Leung was wearing a heavy wool jacket, long wool socks and a wool hat, and his knees were covered with wool leg warmers. Despite all his added clothing, Mr. Leung was still cold.

Consumption of large quantities of tonifying herbs helped only slightly; Mr. Leung still felt as though his body was air conditioned from the spine inward.

First I treated LI-4, GB-20, GV-14, BL-12, and BL-13. Then I applied 7 red bean size direct moxa to GV-14. The next day, Mr. Leung felt that his back was much warmer. For the second treatment I applied 5 direct moxa on BL-13 and 5 direct moxa on GV-20. When I visited the patient on the third day, I noticed that he had removed his wool hat, and that the upper part of his body felt warm. On the fourth day, I applied 10 direct moxa to GV-3, and five direct moxa to CV-6 and CV-4. On the fifth day, I applied 5 red bean size direct moxa to BL-23 and GB-31. The lower part of his body and his legs now felt much warmer.

On the sixth day, I applied 7 direct moxa to the points called "Eyes of the Knees." After this application of moxa, he never found it necessary to wrap his knees again. At this time I also applied 5 direct moxa to ST-36; then his whole body felt warm. Finally, on the seventh day, I applied moxa to GV-4 and again to the Eyes of the Knees. His whole body was both warmer and stronger.

• *Case XVIII: Coldness of the Body with Sha*

Api City, North Borneo, Spring, 1962

Madame Kong, 26 years old, had experienced cold sensations throughout her body for several years. Finally, she made an appointment to see me, and flew the hundred miles from where she lived to Api City for treatment.

Although cold sensations such as this should have been from an overcooling condition, upon examination I found that she also had a considerable amount of *Sha.* Her body was weak from having had this condition, and, although she was a resident of tropical North Borneo, she wore a wool jacket all day, every day.

First, I treated GB-20, GV-14, and BL-12. I applied 5 red bean size moxa to GV-14. The next day she felt no effect from the treatment. Most such cases respond immediately to this treatment, and I was surprised that there wasn't some improvement. Thinking that the lack of effect was due to the fact that the condition had existed for many years, the next day I applied direct moxa to BL-12. The third day arrived, with no improvement. I then applied 7 direct moxa to GV-14 and BL-12. The fourth day came and went with no improvement.

This case seemed very strange to me, and I had her rest for several days. After ten days, her condition remained unchanged. It was then that I discovered that her body contained a great deal of *Sha.* Changing my treatment strategy, I did *gwa sha* over her entire body, dividing this treatment into three parts: the neck and back one day, the chest and abdomen the next, and finally the arms and legs.

Her whole body was dark purple-red as a result of the whole body gwa sha. I directed her not to eat rice, fried foods, or any overheating foods over the next several days. By the fifth day, the *sha* was gone.

I then continued with the moxa treatment that had proved so unsuccessful in the beginning of Madame Kung's treatment. I applied 7 red bean size direct moxa to BL-38, and 3 moxa to ST-36. Now, her whole body became warm, and she was able to shed her heavy garments. This treatment was repeated on the following day.

On the third day, I burned direct moxa on BL-38 and CV-4, and on the fourth day, I applied 5 direct moxa on CV-12 and 10 direct moxa on GV-4. Her whole body was now as warm as could be.

I returned to Api City in 1963. Madame Kong's mother then told me that she was now very healthy.

• *Case XIX: Insomnia Caused by Sha*

North Borneo, February, 1963

Miss Kong, age 19, had great difficulty falling asleep; once asleep, she could only stay asleep for 3 or 4 hours.

I began treatment by needling HT-7 and PC-5, and continued with needles to SP-6, SP-9, and SP-1. Finally, I needled GB-20, GV-16, and BL-13. That night, the patient fell asleep easily. However, several hours after falling asleep she awoke, and could not return to sleep.

The next day, I repeated the treatment, and added 1 sesame seed size moxa to SP-1. Again she fell asleep easily, and although she awoke again in the night, she was able to fall asleep again.

On her third treatment I looked for *sha,* which I discovered on her back. Miss Kong understood what *sha* was, and asked that I not scratch her neck, only her back. That night she slept better than before, but still woke up too early in the morning. On the fourth day, I scratched her neck, without using any needle treatment, and that night she slept a full eight hours.

Following my treatments of Miss Kong, I left Borneo for Hong Kong. After several months, her mother wrote to say that her daughter was still able to sleep normally, and was now able to study without difficulty.

• *Case XX: Treatment of a Seven Year Old Case of Clenched Fingers*

Hong Kong, Summer, 1946

Mr. Lai was 18 years old when he came from Canton to Hong Kong to see me for treatment. Eight years ago, he told me, the ring finger on his right hand suddenly bent inward of its own volition. To stretch this finger, he had to apply force with his other hand. He told his parents of his condition, but they did nothing to help him. Day by day, another finger — first the pointing finger, then the middle finger, the little finger and finally the thumb — bent inward as the ring finger had done. Now, there was no way to stretch them with his other hand. This had all occurred during the Japanese occupation of Canton, a time when it was difficult to find a good doctor. When the war was over in 1946, his father brought him to Hong Kong for treatment. However, none of the doctors to whom he was brought could help. Finally, he was brought to see me.

First, I treated LU-5, PC-3, and PC-5, and obtained a stimulus down to the fingers. Then I treated PC-7, sending the stimulus to all three of the middle fingers. Then I needled HT-7 to stimulate the small finger. Next, I needled LI-5 and LI-4 to stimulate the thumb.

After the needles, I burned 5 green bean size moxa on PC-3, PC-5, and PC-6, treating one point each day for three days. After three days, all the numbness was gone, and Mr. Lee could stretch his pointing finger and middle finger. After 7 treatments, the small finger and the thumb could be stretched. After 14 treatments, the ring finger could be stretched. The patient returned to Canton, completely recovered.

• *Case XXI: A Case of Flatulence*

Hong Kong, November, 1958

An eleven year old boy of the Leung family was growing more and more emaciated every day. His father took him to the medical doctor, whose diagnosis was abdominal worms. The vermifuge prescribed, however, proved to be ineffective, and the boy entered the local hospital, where his condition continued to deteriorate. His entire abdomen was bloated with gas.

When the boy came to see me, his upper and lower abdomen were filled with air. His rib bones and iliac crest were indistinguishable from the swelling. His breathing was shallow, and he was anorexic.

I began treatment by needling LI-4, PC-6, then ST-36, and SP-6, followed by CV-13, CV-12, and CV-10. At last, I treated ST-25, CV-6 and CV-4. After needling, I used indirect moxa with the moxa instrument on all the abdominal points. I also applied 5 direct moxa on CV-12 and CV-6.

That night, the boy experienced a lot of belching and flatulence, and the following morning, his abdomen was smaller. In addition, he felt less full and had something of an appetite. I then repeated the treatment just given, and added direct moxa on CV-13 and CV-4. That night, more gas was released from the boy's abdomen by belching and flatulating.

On the third day, I applied direct moxa on CV-10 and ST-36. After seven treatments, the boy was completely recovered.

• *Case XXII: Treatment of First-Stage Uterine Cancer*

Hong Kong, November, 1955

At the beginning of her disease, Mrs. Cheung, 30 years old, had been experiencing irregular menstruation. Each month, she bled several times, accompanied by discharges. She felt that her abdomen was tight and filled up, and that her whole body was tired. She was too fatigued to do anything, even to talk, and her appetite was poor. When she finally went into the government hospital, she was diagnosed as having uterine cancer in its first stages. Although medical science still does not know the cause of cancer, the old Chinese medical books say that it comes from depression and sorrow, which inhibit the body's circulation.

Because of hospital overcrowding, Mrs. Cheung was told that her surgery could not be scheduled for some time. After two months of waiting, she called me and asked if I could help her. I remembered Mrs. Cheung from having treated her son for a carbuncle some time ago.

On the first day, I treated LI-4, SP-6, CV-6, CV-4, ST-25, ST-29, and GB-26 on the left side of the abdomen. Then I used indirect moxa on ST-25, CV-6, CV-4, and GB-26.

The next day, the patient said that she felt much better, and had slept quite well that night. I then treated the same points as on the first day, with the addition of 7 direct moxa (1/2 rice grain size) on the left Tu Yin. On the third day, the full feeling in her abdomen was gone, and her abdomen felt much softer. This day, I repeated the past treatments, with the modification of burning the moxa on Tu Yin of the right side rather than the left. On the fourth day, I again repeated the past treatments, and burned moxa on Tu Yin bilaterally.

On the fifth and sixth days, I applied needles to BL-23 bilaterally along with the treatment mentioned above. I also applied 5 green bean size moxa to GB-26 on the left side. By this time, all vaginal discharges had ceased.

On the seventh, eighth, and ninth treatments, I added red bean size direct moxa to CV-3. On the tenth and eleventh treatments, I applied moxa to CV-4. On the twelfth day, I applied fourteen red bean size moxa to Pee Gun. After these treatments, the patient felt much better.

After several months, Mrs. Cheung returned to see me with new patients for me to treat. She herself felt normal and healthy, and did not stay to be treated, but left to visit her mother.

• *Case XXIII: Jumping up of Both Legs*

Hong Kong, Summer, 1964

When he came to see me, Mr. Chang, 51, had been having his sleep interrupted by uncontrollable jumping of his legs when he lay down.

First I needled GB-34a, GB-39 and BL-18. Then I applied 3 red bean size moxa on GB-34a. The next day, the jumping was much less. That day, I repeated the treatment, and by the third day, his legs jumped up only 2 or 3 times, whereas before they would jump as much as 10 times.

On the third day, I applied moxa to GB-39, and on the fourth day, I only used a needle there, since the previous night Mr. Chang's legs had not jumped at all.

Commentary: The nerves are controlled by the liver, and are said to meet at GB-34. I used GB-34a in this patient because the point was reactive, i.e. he experienced soreness there. The gallbladder meridian is associated with the liver meridian, and treating gallbladder points benefits the liver.

• *Case XXIV: A Boy with Weakened Knees*

Sarawak, May, 1963

When the nine year old Wong boy came to see me, his knees were so weak that he could not straighten them enough to walk; unless he held on to them, he was able only to kneel down.

I first needled Eyes of the Knees. Then I applied 5 green bean size moxa on those points and to Hok Deng on both sides. Throughout the entire treatment, which involved the burning of 30 direct moxa, the young boy did not cry, devoted as he was to getting better.

After the treatment, I asked the boy to stand up and walk so that I could gauge the effectiveness of the treatment. He was able to stand up straight, and walked around the house several times normally. His mother was overjoyed, and all the other patients waiting for their treatments cheered. As a result of this single treatment, young Wong was completely cured.

• *Case XXV: Acute Inflammation with Mucus in the Knee (Crane's Knee)*

Hong Kong, Summer, 1949

Due to an accident in which he had fallen and injured his knee, the six year old Ng boy came to see me with his left knee red and swollen to twice its normal size, bent to a 45° angle and extremely painful. Western medical doctors were unable to help his condition.

On the first visit, I needled BL-54, ST-33, SP-10, Eyes of the Knee, SP-9, ST-36 on the left side, and GB-34. After this treatment, the patient was in less pain and was able to sleep much better. The next day I repeated the same treatment, this time including 5 direct green bean size moxa on Eyes of the Knees. The boy's father was not optimistic about a cure for his son, and believed that the nerves had become permanently shortened.

On the third day, I applied 3 direct moxa on ST-33 and SP-10 as well as needling the above points. On the fourth day, I added to the above points 3 red bean size moxa on SP-9 and GB-34. Now, although the boy did not feel much pain, the knee was still quite swollen. On the fifth day, I applied electricity to the needles inserted into Eyes of the Knee for five minutes. The next day, the knee was much less swollen.

After this, I use electricity on Eyes of the Knee every day, while applying direct moxa to all the knee points at three different times: the first group treated with moxa was ST-33 and SP-10; the second group was Eyes of the Knee; the third group GB-34 and SP-9. This was done every day for two weeks, alternating groups each day, and using electricity on Eyes of the Knee at each treatment. After these two weeks, the boy was completely recovered.

I met this boy and his father at a wedding party five years later. The boy had grown very tall, and was free of knee problems.

• *Case XXVI: Dropping Down of the Patella*

Hong Kong, Spring, 1964

The four year old girl of the Lim family had had a fever three years ago that changed into polio. When she came to see me, she was unable to walk on her right leg because the patella had become dislodged, and had fallen to the right side of the knee area. She had come to see me to be treated for her polio, but a case that has lasted three years is very difficult to treat.

Even though the patella was misplaced, I located the point Hok Deng on it, and burned 5 direct moxa on it. When the girl returned the next day, it was found that the patella had moved upward, and that the moxa scar on her skin was below he Hok Deng crease. I then applied moxa on the new Hok Deng point. By the third day, the patella had return to its normal position. Finally, I repeated the procedure one last time, to secure the position of the bone. The child was able to start walking.

Note: Hok Deng is located in the center of the patella, not on the upper edge of the patella as presented in some books.

• *Case XXVII: An Allergic Reaction to Antibiotic*

Hong Kong, Autumn, 1958

Mr. Sheck, an acupuncture student, had taken a sulfa drug several days before coming to see me, and had broken out into hives, with intense itching. Using the procedure to check for sympathetic nerve imbalance, I found every meridian normal except for the spleen meridian. SP-1 on the left side withstood 10 seconds of heat application; SP-1 on the right withstood 30 seconds. I therefore needled BL-20 on the left, and applied 3 green bean size moxa the right. After this treatment, the itching ceased and the hives were gone. After eight years, there has been no recurrence of this problem.

Index

The index has been organized in three sections. The **General Index,** which follows immediately, includes references to the conditions, treatments, techniques, and concepts discussed in the text. A **List of Prescriptions**, indexed alphabetically by condition, begins on page 374. The final section, the **Volume I Point Reference**, beginning on page 375, cross references all the acupoints to **The Book of Acupuncture Points**, Volume One of **A Complete Course in Acupuncture**, where the information regarding specific location, stimulation, technique, and other point effects may be found. Included are the section number, illustration number, and page number for each acupoint ordered by meridian.

Abdomen

Asthma

Cramp

Diagnosis

Diagnosis, continued

Diarrhea

Direct Moxa

Direct Moxa, continued

Ear

Eye

Fever

Infant

Inflammation

Intestine

Kidneys

Neck

Needles

Pain

Paralysis

Pulse

Pulse, continued

Sha

Stomach

Tongue

Urine

Vomiting

List of Prescriptions

Herbal formulae are presented in the text for the following conditions.

Volume I Point Reference

All entries in this section follow the format of point number followed by the section number, illustration number and page number of the reference in **The Book of Acupuncture Points**, Volume One of this set.

Bladder Meridian

Point; Sec; Ilus; Page

BL-1; 6,4; 8; 26
BL-2; 6,2; 8; 25
BL-3; 42,1; 236
BL-4; 42,2; 236
BL-5; 42,3; 236
BL-6; 42,4; 237
BL-7; 42,5; 237
BL-8; 42,6; 238
BL-9; 42,7; 238
BL-10; 4,3; 6; 18
BL-11; 17,1; 19; 82
BL-12; 17,2; 19; 83
BL-13; 17,3; 19; 83
BL-14; 42,8; 238
BL-15; 17,4; 19; 84
BL-16; 42,9; 239
BL-17; 17,5; 19; 84
BL-18; 17,6; 19; 85
BL-19; 17,7; 19; 85
BL-20; 17,8; 19; 86
BL-21; 17,9; 19; 86
BL-22; 17,10; 19; 87
BL-23; 17,11; 19; 88
BL-24; 42,10; 239
BL-25; 17,12; 19; 89
BL-26; 42,11; 239
BL-27; 17,13; 19; 89
BL-28; 17,14; 19; 90
BL-29; 42,12; 240
BL-30; 17,15; 19; 90
BL-31; 17,16; 19; 91
BL-32; 17,17; 19; 91
BL-33; 17,18; 19; 92
BL-34; 17,19; 19; 92
BL-35; 17,20; 19; 93
BL-36; 42,13; 240
BL-37; 42,14; 241
BL-38; 18,1; 20; 95
BL-39; 42,15; 241
BL-40; 42,16; 241
BL-41; 42,17; 242
BL-42; 42,18; 242
BL-43; 42,19; 242
BL-44; 42,20; 243
BL-45; 42,21; 243
BL-46; 42,22; 243
BL-47; 18,3; 20; 97
BL-48; 42,23; 244
BL-49; 42,24; 244
BL-50; 27,1; 29; 155
BL-51; 42,25; 244
BL-52; 42,26; 245
BL-53; 42,27; 245
BL-54; 27,2; 29; 155
BL-55; 42,28; 245
BL-56; 42,29; 246
BL-57; 27,3; 29; 157
BL-58; 42,30; 246
BL-59; 42,31; 247
BL-60; 27,5; 29; 158
BL-61; 42,32; 247
BL-62; 27,6; 29; 158
BL-63; 27,7; 29; 159
BL-64; 42,33; 248
BL-65; 42,34; 249
BL-66; 42,35; 249
BL-67; 27,8; 29; 159

Conception Vessel Meridian

Point; Sec; Ilus; Page

CV-1; 13,7; 15; 62
CV-2; 13,6; 15; 62
CV-3; 13,5; 15; 61
CV-4; 13,4; 15; 60
CV-5; 13,3; 15; 59
CV-6; 13,2; 15; 58
CV-7; 13,1; 15; 57
CV-8; 12,8; 14; 55
CV-9; 12,7; 14; 54
CV-10; 12,6; 14; 54
CV-11; 12,5; 14; 53
CV-12; 12,4; 14; 53
CV-13; 12,3; 14; 52

CV-14; 12,2; 14; 52
CV-15; 12,1; 14; 51
CV-16; 10,4; 12; 43
CV-17; 10,3; 12; 43
CV-18; 29,1; 169
CV-19; 29,2; 169
CV-20; 29,3; 170
CV-21; 29,4; 170
CV-22; 10,2; 12; 42
CV-23; 10,1; 12; 41
CV-24; 8,3; 10; 32

Gallbladder Meridian

Point; Sec; Ilus; Page

GB-1; 6,5; 8; 27
GB-2; 5,2; 7; 21
GB-3; 41,1; 224
GB-4; 41,2; 224
GB-5; 41,3; 225
GB-6; 41,4; 225
GB-7; 41,5; 226
GB-8; 41,6; 226
GB-9; 41,7; 226
GB-10; 41,8; 227
GB-11; 41,9; 227
GB-12; 41,10; 228
GB-13; 3,1; 6; 16
GB-14; 6,1; 8; 25
GB-15; 2,1; 5; 14
GB-16; 2,2; 5; 14
GB-17; 41,11; 228
GB-18; 41,12; 228
GB-19; 41,13; 229
GB-20; 4,4; 6; 19
GB-21; 15,1; 17; 71
GB-22; 41,14; 229
GB-23; 41,15; 230
GB-24; 41,16; 230
GB-25; 41,17; 231
GB-26; 11,7; 13; 49
GB-27; 41,18; 231
GB-28; 41,19; 232
GB-29; 41,20; 232
GB-30; 28,1; 30; 161
GB-31; 28,3; 30; 162
GB-32; 41,21; 232
GB-33; 28,4; 30; 162
GB-34; 28,5; 30; 163
GB-35; 41,22; 233
GB-36; 41,23; 233
GB-37; 41,24; 234
GB-38; 28,6; 30; 163
GB-39; 28,7; 30; 164
GB-40; 28,8; 30; 164
GB-41; 41,25; 234
GB-42; 41,26; 235
GB-43; 41,27; 235
GB-44; 28,9; 30; 165

Governing Vessel Meridian

Point; Sec; Ilus; Page

GV-1; 16,10; 18; 80
GV-2; 16,9; 18; 79
GV-3; 16,8; 18; 79
GV-4; 16,7; 18; 78
GV-5; 30,1; 171
GV-6; 30,2; 171
GV-7; 30,3; 171
GV-8; 30,4; 172
GV-9; 16,6; 18; 77
GV-10; 16,5; 18; 77
GV-11; 16,4; 18; 76
GV-12; 16,3; 18; 76
GV-13; 16,2; 18; 75
GV-14; 16,1; 18; 74
GV-15; 4,2; 6; 18
GV-16; 4,1; 6; 17
GV-17; 30,5; 172
GV-18; 30,6; 172
GV-19; 1,6; 5; 13
GV-20; 1,5; 5; 13
GV-21; 1,4; 5; 12
GV-22; 1,3; 5; 12
GV-23; 1,2; 5; 11
GV-24; 1,1; 5; 11
GV-25; 7,1; 9; 29
GV-26; 8,1; 10; 31
GV-27; 30,7; 173
GV-28; 30,8; 173

Heart Meridian

Point; Sec; Ilus; Page

HT-1; 32,1; 177
HT-2; 32,2; 177
HT-3; 19,14; 21; 108
HT-4; 19,15; 21; 109
HT-5; 19,16; 21; 109
HT-6; 19,17; 21; 110
HT-7; 19,18; 21; 111
HT-8; 19,19; 21; 112
HT-9; 19,20; 21; 113

Kidney Meridian

Point; Sec; Ilus; Page

KI-1; 25,1; 27; 141
KI-2; 25,2; 27; 142
KI-3; 25,3; 27; 143
KI-4; 25,5; 27; 145
KI-5; 37,1; 196
KI-6; 25,4; 27; 144
KI-7; 25,6; 27; 145
KI-8; 25,7; 27; 146
KI-9; 37,2; 196
KI-10; 37,3; 197
KI-11; 37,4; 197
KI-12; 37,5; 198
KI-13; 37,6; 198
KI-14; 37,7; 198
KI-15; 37,8; 199
KI-16; 37,9; 199
KI-17; 37,10; 199
KI-18; 37,11; 200
KI-19; 37,12; 200
KI-20; 37,13; 200
KI-21; 37,14; 201
KI-22; 37,15; 201
KI-23; 37,16; 201
KI-24; 37,17; 202
KI-25; 37,18; 202
KI-26; 37,19; 202
KI-27; 37,20; 203

Large Intestine Meridian

Point; Sec; Ilus; Page

LI-1; 20,1; 22; 115
LI-2; 34,1; 179
LI-3; 34,2; 179
LI-4; 20,2; 22; 115
LI-5; 20,3; 22; 116
LI-6; 34,3; 180
LI-7; 34,4; 180
LI-8; 34,5; 181
LI-9; 34,6; 181
LI-10; 20,4; 22; 117
LI-11; 20,5; 22; 118
LI-12; 34,7; 182
LI-13; 20,6; 22; 119
LI-14; 20,7; 22; 119
LI-15; 15,2; 17; 72
LI-16; 15,3; 17; 72
LI-17; 34,8; 183
LI-18; 34,9; 183
LI-19; 34,10; 184
LI-20; 7,2; 9; 29

Lung Meridian

Point; Sec; Ilus; Page

LU-1; 11,5; 13; 47
LU-2; 31,1; 174
LU-3; 31,2; 174
LU-4; 31,3; 175
LU-5; 19,1; 21; 99
LU-6; 31,4; 175
LU-7; 19,2; 21; 100
LU-8; 19,3; 21; 101
LU-9; 19,4; 21; 101
LU-10; 31,5; 176
LU-11; 19,5; 21; 102

Liver Meridian

Point; Sec; Ilus; Page

LV-1; 24,1; 26; 137
LV-2; 24,2; 26; 137
LV-3; 24,3; 26; 138
LV-4; 24,4; 26; 138
LV-5; 39,1; 211
LV-6; 39,2; 211
LV-7; 24,5; 26; 139
LV-8; 24,6; 26; 139
LV-9; 39,3; 212
LV-10; 39,4; 212
LV-11; 14,6; 16; 69
LV-12; 39,5; 212
LV-13; 11,6; 13; 48
LV-14; 11,4; 13; 46

Pericardium Meridian

Point; Sec; Ilus; Page

PC-1; 33,1; 178
PC-2; 33,2; 178
PC-3; 19,6; 21; 103
PC-4; 19,7; 21; 103
PC-5; 19,9; 21; 104
PC-6; 19,10; 21; 105
PC-7; 19,11; 21; 105
PC-8; 21; 106;
PC-9; 19,13; 21; 107

Small Intestine Meridian

Point; Sec; Ilus; Page

SI-1; 22,1; 24; 125
SI-2; 36,1; 191
SI-3; 22,2; 24; 125
SI-4; 22,3; 24; 126
SI-5; 22,4; 24; 126
SI-6; 36,2; 191
SI-7; 36,3; 192
SI-8; 22,5; 24; 127
SI-9; 36,4; 192
SI-10; 36,5; 192
SI-11; 36,6; 193
SI-12; 36,7; 193
SI-13; 36,8; 193
SI-14; 36,9; 194
SI-15; 36,10; 194
SI-16; 36,11; 194
SI-17; 36,12; 195
SI-18; 36,13; 195
SI-19; 5,3; 7; 22

Spleen Meridian

Point; Sec; Ilus; Page

SP-1; 23,1; 25; 132
SP-2; 23,2; 25; 132
SP-3; 38,1; 204
SP-4; 23,3; 25; 133
SP-5; 23,4; 25; 133
SP-6; 23,5; 25; 134
SP-7; 38,2; 204
SP-8; 38,3; 205
SP-9; 23,6; 25; 135
SP-10; 23,7; 25; 135
SP-11; 38,4; 205
SP-12; 38,5; 206
SP-13; 38,6; 206
SP-14; 38,7; 207
SP-15; 38,8; 207
SP-16; 38,9; 208
SP-17; 38,10; 208
SP-18; 38,11; 209
SP-19; 38,12; 209
SP-20; 38,13; 210
SP-21; 38,14; 210

Stomach Meridian

Point; Sec; Ilus; Page

ST-1; 40,1; 213
ST-2; 40,2; 213
ST-3; 40,3; 214
ST-4; 8,2; 10; 31
ST-5; 40,4; 214
ST-6; 5,5; 7; 23
ST-7; 40,5; 215
ST-8; 3,2; 6; 16
ST-9; 40,6; 215
ST-10; 40,7; 216
ST-11; 40,8; 216
ST-12; 11,1; 13; 45
ST-13; 40,9; 216
ST-14; 40,10; 217
ST-15; 40,11; 217
ST-16; 11,2; 13; 45
ST-18; 11,3; 13; 46
ST-19; 40,12; 217
ST-20; 40,13; 218
ST-21; 40,14; 218
ST-22; 40,15; 218
ST-23; 40,16; 219
ST-24; 40,17; 219
ST-25; 14,1; 16; 66
ST-26; 40,18; 219
ST-27; 14,2; 16; 67
ST-28; 14,3; 16; 67
ST-29; 14,4; 16; 68
ST-30; 14,5; 16; 68
ST-31; 40,19; 220
ST-32; 40,20; 220
ST-33; 26,1; 28; 148
ST-34; 40,21; 220
ST-35; 40,22; 221
ST-36a; 26,6; 28; 150
ST-36; 26,5; 28; 150
ST-37; 40,23; 221
ST-38; 40,24; 222
ST-39; 40,25; 222
ST-40; 26,7; 28; 151
ST-41; 26,8; 28; 151
ST-42; 26,9; 28; 152
ST-43; 40,26; 223
ST-44; 26,10; 28; 152
ST-45; 26,11; 28; 153

Triple Warmer Meridian

Point; Sec; Ilus; Page

Extra Points

Point; Sec; Ilus; Page